Obstetrics and Gynaecology for Finals, DRCOG and MRCOG

Obstetrics and Gynaecology for Finals, DRCOG and MRCOG
A REVISION GUIDE

JANICE RYMER
Professor of Obstetrics and Gynaecology,
King's College London School of Medicine
Honorary Consultant Gynaecologist,
Guy's and St Thomas' Hospital Trust

and

NORMAN SMITH
Consultant Obstetrician
Honorary Clinical Senior Lecturer
Aberdeen Maternity Hospital

Radcliffe Publishing
Oxford • New York

Radcliffe Publishing Ltd
18 Marcham Road
Abingdon
Oxon OX14 1AA
United Kingdom

www.radcliffe-oxford.com
Electronic catalogue and worldwide online ordering facility.

British Library Cataloguing in Publication Data

A catalogue record for this book is available from the British Library.

ISBN-13: 978 1 84619 0 735

Typeset by Pindar NZ, Auckland, New Zealand
Printed and bound by TJI Digital, Padstow, Cornwall, UK

Contents

Preface

This book is intended to test knowledge in obstetrics and gynaecology at all levels from undergraduate to postgraduate. It covers most aspects of obstetrics and gynaecology, and all questions have comprehensive answers to act as a learning aid. The best of five questions and answers are targeted for those sitting the DRCOG, the multiple-choice questions for both DRCOG and MRCOG and the extended matching questions for those sitting MRCOG. However, all those who wish to advance their knowledge will find this book useful, and undergraduates will be delighted, as the book covers all types of questions that they are likely to encounter as modern written examination methods move away from essays and short-answer questions into best of fives and EMQs.

Janice Rymer
Norman Smith
January 2009

About the authors

Professor Janice Rymer is Professor of Obstetrics and Gynaecology at King's College London School of Medicine and Honorary Consultant Gynaecologist at Guy's and St Thomas' Hospital Trust. She has been on the DRCOG examination committee, chaired the MRCOG OSCE committee and examined for DRCOG, MRCOG and undergraduate examinations.

Dr Norman Smith is a Consultant Obstetrician and Honorary Clinical Senior Lecturer at Aberdeen Maternity Hospital. He has examined for the DRCOG, been a member of the RCOG OSCE subcommittee and MCQ subcommittee and regularly examines for the MRCOG as well as undergraduate examinations.

Together Dr Smith and Professor Rymer have organised MRCOG courses at the Royal College of Obstetricians and Gynaecologists and internationally. They both have vast experience in small and large group teaching and in setting, examining and marking undergraduate and postgraduate examinations. They are both actively involved in clinical work and clinical teaching and regularly contribute to education courses.

Acknowledgements

We would like to acknowledge images kindly given to us from Alison Smith, Senior Ultrasonographer at Guy's and St Thomas' Hospital NHS Foundation Trust.

Multiple-choice questions: Paper 1

1   Natural menopause:
    a   may occur under the age of 30
    b   is associated with an increase in HDL cholesterol
    c   accelerates bone loss
    d   causes an increase in the karyopyknotic index (KPI)
    e   occurs at an average age of 54 in the UK.

2   Secondary amenorrhoea may be due to:
    a   thyrotoxicosis
    b   virilising ovarian tumour
    c   imperforate hymen
    d   Asherman's syndrome
    e   endometriosis.

3   Regarding human fertility.
    a   Fertilisation usually occurs five to seven days before
        implantation.
    b   Subfertility is common following mumps in women.
    c   An adverse male factor is detectable in about 30% of couples
        with low fertility.
    d   Hyperstimulation syndrome may occur as a complication of
        clomid therapy.
    e   Testicular biopsy may be used in the investigation of
        azoospermia.

4 Sterilisation:
  a in men has a failure rate of about 1 in 300 cases
  b prevents pregnancy in a similar order of magnitude to the Mirena levonorgestrel intrauterine system
  c when it fails can be associated with an ectopic pregnancy
  d in women decreases menstrual loss
  e in women can be successfully reversed if clips were used for the original operation in >80% of cases.

5 Regarding thromboembolic disease.
  a There is a greater risk in a multiple than in a singleton pregnancy.
  b Heparin should not be given in the first trimester.
  c Warfarin increases the likelihood of fetal haemorrhage.
  d In pregnancy heparin therapy can cause maternal osteoporosis.
  e The risk is increased in women who are blood group O.

6 Monozygotic twins:
  a are less common than dizygotic twins
  b are commonly familial
  c may be reliably distinguished from dizygotic twins by the naked-eye examination of the fetal membranes and placentae
  d have a higher incidence of placenta praevia than singleton pregnancies
  e are associated with acute polyhydramnios.

7 Spina bifida:
  a is associated with raised maternal serum α-fetoprotein (AFP) levels
  b can be diagnosed by ultrasound scan during the third trimester
  c is inherited as an autosomal recessive
  d is associated with dilated cerebral ventricles
  e screening may be tested with maternal serum.

8 In development of the female genital tract:
  a the fallopian tubes are derived from the Müllerian ducts

b the external genitalia can be recognised as male or female by the 16th week of fetal life

c failure of fusion of the Müllerian ducts results in a double uterus

d the upper third of the vagina is formed from the cloaca

e Wolffian ducts degenerate in the absence of a Y chromosome.

9 In human genetics:
a an XO genotype is associated with male somatotype
b the total number of chromosomes in both males and females is 48
c chromatin-positive cells (Barr body present) are characteristic of normal women
d first-trimester chorionic villus sampling is associated with a fetal loss of 1%
e the Y chromosome determines the development of the ovary.

10 In the normal cervix:
a the canal is lined by the transitional epithelium
b the mucus is scanty at the time of ovulation
c the level of the squamo-columnar junction varies at different phases of reproductive life
d keratinised stratified epithelium is found over the vaginal aspects of the cervix
e the squamo-columnar junction is usually visible on speculum examination after menopause.

11 In the fetal skull:
a the biparietal diameter is approximately 9.5 cm at the term
b the lambdoidal suture runs between the frontal and parietal bones
c the bregma is the area lying between the parietal and occipital bones
d the sub-occipito bregmatic diameter is the engaging diameter when the head is fully flexed in a vertex presentation
e the occiput is the denominator in a vertex presentation.

12 In the fetal circulatory system:
   a blood flows from the fetus to the placenta in the umbilical
      arteries
   b the ductus arteriosus closes during labour
   c placental circulation starts at about one week after
      implantation
   d the heart becomes a four-chamber organ at about seven
      weeks' gestational age
   e reversed end diastolic flow in the umbilical artery is associated
      with fetal hypoxia.

13 The following hormones are secreted within the posterior lobe
    of the human pituitary gland:
   a oxytocin
   b thyroid-stimulating hormone
   c luteinising hormone
   d adrenocorticotrophin
   e prolactin.

14 Regarding ovum and spermatozoa.
   a The spermatozoa are responsible for approximately 10% of
      the volume of the ejaculate.
   b The fertilised ovum can be fertilised up to four days after
      ovulation.
   c Human spermatozoa are capable of fertilising an oocyte when
      aspirated from the testis.
   d Human spermatozoa when mature have undergone a
      reduction division of their nucleus.
   e The fertilised ovum implants at the 16 cell stage

15 Regarding miscarriage.
   a If recurrent, it can be associated with parental chromosomal
      translocation.
   b If recurrent, it can be associated with sickle cell trait.
   c The clinical diagnosis of incomplete miscarriage is assisted by
      digital examination of the cervical canal.
   d Cervical incompetence causes recurrent first-trimester
      miscarriage.

    e Missed miscarriage should be suspected if the uterine size is greater than expected for gestational age.

16 Circulatory changes in a healthy woman during a normal pregnancy include:
    a a significant rise in cardiac output only during the second and third trimesters
    b a reduction in tidal volume
    c an increase in glomerular filtration rate
    d a reduction in peripheral blood flow
    e a uterine blood flow at term of the order of 200 mL/minute.

17 Termination of pregnancy:
    a is illegal after 20 weeks' gestation
    b after 16 weeks is most safely achieved by hysterotomy
    c requires the signature of two gynaecologists
    d can be achieved by the intra-amniotic administration of prostaglandin
    e complications include infertility in about 2% of cases.

18 In ectopic pregnancy:
    a the gestation sac is within the fallopian tube
    b the diagnosis can be excluded by ultrasound
    c β-HCG levels are usually detectable in a concentrated urinary sample
    d there may be a coexistent intrauterine pregnancy
    e the patient may present with brown vaginal discharge.

19 Hypertension in pregnancy:
    a is of little significance unless accompanied by proteinuria
    b causes fetal growth restriction in more than half of affected women
    c is associated with an increased incidence of bleeding from placental praevia
    d should be assessed by admission to hospital
    e is a contraindication to the use of intramuscular Syntometrine.

20 In pre-eclampsia:
   a the perinatal mortality is raised
   b epigastric pain may indicate impending eclampsia
   c there are lowered serum urate levels
   d there may be no fetus
   e the liquor volume may be diminished.

21 A diagnosis of severe dyskaryosis taken on a cervical smear during pregnancy:
   a may have been confused with the normal cytological changes of pregnancy
   b is more likely to indicate an adenocarcinoma rather than CIN 3
   c is investigated by colposcopically directed biopsy postnatally
   d is a contraindication to intercourse
   e is an indication for delivery by Caesarean section.

22 Insulin-dependent diabetes mellitus in pregnancy:
   a is associated with an increased risk of congenital abnormality
   b reduces maternal insulin requirements
   c is best monitored by measuring glycosylated haemoglobin levels
   d should be taken into consideration when interpreting the serum screening for Down's syndrome
   e can be associated with fetal growth restriction.

23 Heavy menstrual bleeding can be treated with:
   a the combined oral contraceptive pill
   b tranexamic acid
   c medicated intrauterine devices
   d ethamsylate, taken during menstruation
   e mefenamic acid, taken days 19 to 26 of the cycle.

24 Dysmenorrhoea:
   a can be successfully treated with non-steroidal anti-inflammatory drugs
   b can be caused by anovulation

c   is more severe with a retroverted uterus

d   can be caused by endometriosis

e   can be caused by anterior vaginal wall prolapse.

25 The progesterone-only pill:

a   is a recognised cause of secondary amenorrhoea

b   can be safely given to lactating women and before recommencing menstruation

c   should not be prescribed to an individual with a history of a deep venous thrombosis

d   acts mainly by inhibiting ovulation

e   increases tubal motility.

26 The intrauterine contraceptive device:

a   carries at least a 1 in 8 chance of expulsion

b   contains copper as a means of reducing endometrial receptivity to implantation

c   increases the risk of miscarriage should pregnancy occur

d   is contraindicated with a past history of ectopic pregnancies

e   significantly increases the risk of fetal abnormality should pregnancy occur.

27 Epidurals sited during labour:

a   require pre-loading with fluid

b   are contraindicated when a coagulation defect is present

c   lower the maternal blood pressure

d   decrease the rate of forceps deliveries

e   may be combined deliberately with a spinal anaesthetic.

28 Induction of labour:

a   can be achieved by amniotomy

b   is easiest when the cervix is in a posterior position

c   could be achieved by an ergometrine infusion

d   is indicated with an uncomplicated dichorionic twin pregnancy of greater than 36 weeks' gestation

e   can be achieved by prostaglandin infusion.

29 Delay in the first stage of labour may be caused by:
  a a fractured coccyx
  b cephalopelvic disproportion
  c maternal anaemia
  d a brow presentation
  e dehiscence of a caesarean section scar.

30 Delay in the second stage of labour may be caused by:
  a a rigid perineum
  b a short umbilical cord
  c cervical stenosis following a knife cone biopsy
  d an effective epidural
  e maternal exhaustion.

Answers: MCQs Paper 1

1 a *T* Premature ovarian failure occurs in less than 1% of women under 40 and has a variety of causes including genetic, autoimmune, infective, iatrogenic and idiopathic.

   b *F* When ovarian failure occurs there is a *decrease* in HDL.

   c *T* After ovarian failure there is an additional effect over and above that of age-related bone loss.

   d *F* The KPI is the ratio of superficial cells to parabasal cells. Women in the reproductive age group have a high KPI (estrogenic stimulation gives rise to a higher number of superficial cells). Prepubertal and postmenopausal women have a very low KPI.

   e *F* The average age of menopause in the UK is 50 years, 9 months.

2 a *T* Abnormalities of thyroid function can produce a variety of menstrual disturbances.

   b *T* These tumours are rare (<1% of ovarian tumours) and may present with physical signs of virilisation and genital or breast atrophy as well as menstrual disturbances.

   c *F* Imperforate hymen is associated with *primary* amenorrhoea.

   d *T* Over-vigorous curettage of the endometrial cavity, especially in the presence of infection, may cause scarring and obliteration of the cavity, with subsequent amenorrhoea.

   e *F* Endometriosis is associated with pelvic pain, dyspareunia and dysmenorrhoea, not secondary amenorrhoea.

3 a *T* Sperm and egg fuse in the fimbrial/ampullary end of the fallopian tube and transport between this region and implantation in the endometrium takes between five and seven days.

   b *F* Oophoritis is a very *uncommon* complication of mumps in the female.

   c *T* In broad terms infertility can be categorised as being 30% male factor, 30% female factor and 30% combined factors.

d *T* Yes rarely, but hyperstimulation is a more common complication when parenteral hormone methods are used to induce multiple ovarian follicles.

e *T* Testicular biopsy may be used to see if any sperm are present in the testis.

4 a *T* It is essential that patients about to undergo male sterilisation are made aware that the failure rate is 1 in 300 cases before giving their consent.

b *T* A Mirena IUS also has the advantage of being more readily reversible.

c *T* The possibility of an ectopic pregnancy should be borne in mind when a woman presents with a positive β-HCG post sterilisation.

d *F* A number of well-controlled studies have shown that there is no change to the volume of menstrual bleeding experienced by women after tubal ligation.

e *F* Success rates vary from surgeon to surgeon, but in general success rates of approximately 50% are quoted. Individual expertise and the use of microsurgical techniques may improve the chances of success.

5 a *T* Multiple gestations exacerbate all the complications of pregnancy.

b *F* As heparin does not cross the placenta, it therefore does not directly affect the fetus and is not known to have teratogenic effects.

c *T* Warfarin crosses the placenta and has been associated with a variety of adverse effects, including an increased risk of fetal intracerebral and retroplacental haemorrhage.

d *T* Long-term therapy of at least 10 000 units per day for three months can cause this complication.

e *F* An increased risk is associated with blood groups *other than* O.

6 a *T* Spontaneous conceptions in European and North American twin births account for 11 per 1000 deliveries; worldwide monozygous twins are present in 3.5 per 1000 births.

b *F* Dizygotic twins are familial.

c *F* Monozygotic twins can be monochorionic and/or monoamniotic. Dizygotic twins are dichorionic and diamniotic.

d *T* The increased size of the placenta in monozygotic twins means that there is a greater chance of some part of it encroaching upon the lower segment.

e *T* The incidence of polyhydramnios increases with multiple pregnancy.

7 a *T* Open neural tube defect is associated with spina bifida and raises maternal α-fetoprotein levels.

b *T* Although routine ultrasound scans are usually performed in the second trimester, spina bifida abnormalities may be diagnosed by ultrasound scans in the third trimester.

c *F* Spina bifida does not follow a single gene mode of inheritance. It is multifactorial.

d *T* Characteristic ultrasonic findings in the fetal head are ventriculomegaly, the 'lemon' and 'banana' sign and a reduced BPD (biparietal diameter) and head circumference. The 'lemon' sign is the appearance of the head circumference and the 'banana' sign is the shape of the cerebellum.

e *T* Serum screening includes α-fetoprotein. The latter can therefore be used to screen for open neural tube defects.

8 a *T* Presence of Müllerian inhibitory factor is required for the normal development of the Wolffian ducts along the male phenotype. In its absence the Müllerian ducts contribute to the female phenotype.

b *T* Fetal sexing can be performed ultrasonographically at this stage, but not with 100% diagnostic accuracy.

c *T* Normal uterine anatomy results from fusion of portions of the Müllerian ducts from both sides and breakdown of the midline septum. Failure of this process can result in a variety of anatomical abnormalities.

d *F* The *lower* third of the vagina is formed from the cloaca.

e *T* The Wolffian duct persists in the presence of a Y chromosome.

9   a   *F*   An XO genotype is associated with *female* somatotype and is termed Turner's syndrome.

     b   *F*   The total number of chromosomes in both males and females is *46*.

     c   *T*   This test relies on the presence of inactivated X chromosome, and can still be seen in males with XXY composition.

     d   *T*   CVS, in expert hands, is associated with a fetal loss in the region of 1% and amniocentesis with a loss in the region of 0.5%.

     e   *F*   In the presence of a Y chromosome, Müllerian inhibitory factor suppresses development of the female genital organs.

10   a   *F*   Transitional epithelium lines the urinary tract.

     b   *F*   At the time of ovulation the mucus is typically clear and profuse.

     c   *T*   The squamo-columnar junction is under hormonal influence and so alters during puberty and the menopause.

     d   *F*   Non-keratinised stratified epithelium lines the vagina and encroaches upon the cervix.

     e   *F*   The squamo-columnar junction usually recedes within the endocervical canal after the menopause.

11   a   *T*   The biparietal diameter gradually enlarges during pregnancy and its ultrasonic measurement assists in pregnancy dating during the later part of the first and the second trimester.

     b   *F*   The lambdoidal suture runs between the parietal, temporal and occipital bones.

     c   *F*   The bregma (also known as the anterior fontanelle) lies between the frontal and parietal bones.

     d   *T*   The sub-occipito bregmatic diameter presents the smallest cephalic dimension for passing through the maternal pelvis.

     e   *T*   Each presentation has a denominator: the chin is the denominator in a face presentation and the sacrum is the denominator in a breech presentation.

12 a *T* This is the reverse of the adult situation. Here the arteries carry the deoxygenated blood.

   b *F* Closure of the ductus anteriosus is a postnatal phenomenon.

   c *T* Primitive placental circulation starts shortly after implantation.

   d *T* As a part of ultrasonic screening to rule out congenital anomalies, visualisation of a four-chamber heart excludes a number of the major cardiac malformations.

   e *T* Ideally forward flow should occur in both systole and diastole during Doppler flow studies of the fetal umbilical arteries.

13 a *T* The posterior lobe of the human pituitary gland secretes oxytocin and vasopressin (ADH).

   b *F* Thyroid-stimulating hormone is secreted from the *anterior* lobe.

   c *F* Luteinising hormone is secreted from the *anterior* lobe.

   d *F* Adrenocorticotrophin is secreted from the *anterior* lobe.

   e *F* Prolactin is secreted from the *anterior* lobe.

14 a *F* The vast majority of ejaculate is composed of secretions added from the various glands in the male reproductive tract – from the seminal vesicles, the prostate, the bulbourethral and urethral glands.

   b *F* There is a 'window' of about 24 hours during which the ovum can be fertilised.

   c *T* Direct semen injection into the human oocyte and fertilisation has been achieved using ICSI (intra-cytoplasmic sperm injection).

   d *T* Human spermatozoa carry 23 chromosomes.

   e *F* The fertilised ovum implants days after fertilisation, well past the 16-cell stage.

15 a *T* Chromosomal translocation in either parent can result in the production of unbalanced gametes and increases the incidence of miscarriage for chromosomal abnormality.

   b *F* Recurrent miscarriage is associated with sickle cell *disease*, not trait.

    c *T* The internal cervical os is open and products of conception may be felt.

    d *F* Cervical incompetence is commonly associated with *second*-trimester recurrent miscarriage.

    e *F* The uterus is more commonly *smaller* than would be expected for gestational age.

16 a *F* The cardiac output rises in the *first* trimester and continues to rise in the second and third, reaching a plateau in the third trimester.

    b *F* Tidal volume *increases*.

    c *T* Glomerular filtration rate (GFR) increases by 55% in early pregnancy and up to 60% in late pregnancy.

    d *F* Peripheral blood flow *increases* and is associated with a fall in peripheral vascular resistance.

    e *F* Uterine blood flow at term is approximately 500 mL/minute.

17 a *F* Termination of pregnancy for social reasons has an upper gestation limit of 24 weeks; however, in the presence of significant fetal abnormality no such upper limit exists.

    b *F* Hysterotomy is rarely used to achieve termination of pregnancy; prostaglandin induction of uterine contractions is a safe and successful method.

    c *F* Termination of pregnancy requires the signature of two independent medical practitioners.

    d *T* Prostaglandin can be given by the vaginal, extra-amniotic, intra-amniotic and intravenous routes.

    e *F* Infertility is a rare complication in termination of pregnancy.

18 a *F* The definition of an ectopic pregnancy is conception outside the uterine cavity, not specifically with the fallopian tube. Other sites include abdominal, cervical and ovarian pregnancies.

    b *T* Ultrasound can detect a viable intrauterine pregnancy and exclude the diagnosis in some cases.

    c *T* Sensitive β-HCG urine tests are nearly always positive in the presence of any pregnancy, including those that are ectopic. They can detect β-HCG in the urine at serum levels of 25–50 international units.

d T The incidence of heterotopic pregnancy in the uterine cavity coexisting with another pregnancy elsewhere is in the region of 1 in 30 000. Incidence is increasing with assisted conception.

e T Some vaginal bleeding, which could be a small quantity of brown discharge or moderate fresh blood, may be present with an ectopic pregnancy.

19 a F Although hypertension in pregnancy can be classified by the presence or absence of proteinuria, events such as cerebrovascular accidents can occur with an elevated blood pressure unaccompanied by proteinuria.

b F Patients with hypertension, medically treated or not, are usually screened to detect fetal growth retardation by serial ultrasound measurement. The majority will have only mild to moderate disease, typically not associated with fetal growth outside the normal range.

c F Hypertension is associated with an increased incidence of placental abruption and associated bleeding.

d F Many cases of hypertension can be successfully managed on an outpatient basis.

e T Ergometrine, given intravenously or intramuscularly postpartum in combination with oxytocin, should be withheld. Oxytocin alone is preferred.

20 a T Perinatal mortality is increased due to a variety of factors, the necessity for preterm delivery being one of the most significant.

b T Epigastric pain, visual disturbances, hyper-reflexia and clonus are all signs of impending eclampsia.

c F Serum urate levels tend to be *elevated* in pre-eclampsia.

d T Pre-eclampsia can occur without a fetus with a hydatidiform mole.

e T Poor placental perfusion and diminished fetal renal perfusion can result in a reduction in liquor production.

21 a *F* Pregnancy does not cause dyskaryotic cell appearances.

b *F* Severe dyskaryosis is more likely to be associated with the histological diagnosis of CIN 3. Adenocarcinoma is associated with glandular cell abnormality and is far less likely.

c *F* A diagnosis of severe dyskaryosis in pregnancy is an indication for an urgent colposcopy assessment by an experienced operator to rule out invasive disease.

d *F* Sexual intercourse has not been shown to have any influence on the progression of severe dyskaryosis.

e *F* Vaginal delivery can be safely and successfully achieved in the presence of severe dyskaryosis.

22 a *T* A variety of congenital abnormalities are associated with diabetes mellitus; most studies have documented a two- to fourfold increase.

b *F* Maternal insulin requirements *increase* progressively during the course of pregnancy.

c *F* Glycosylated haemoglobin (HbAic) levels are indicative of previous three to four weeks' mean glucose levels and are not the best method of monitoring.

d *T* Women with insulin-dependent diabetes mellitus have significantly lower maternal α-fetoprotein and unconjugated oestriol levels when compared with women without diabetes. This information is therefore needed to prevent an excess of false positive triple test results in diabetic women.

e *T* Severe diabetics can have poor placental perfusion resulting in fetal growth retardation.

23 a *T* The combined oral contraceptive pill reduces menstrual blood loss by an average of 50%.

b *T* The antifibrinolytic tranexamic acid is taken for the duration of the menses and is associated with a reduction in blood loss in the region of 50%.

c *T* Intrauterine devices which release small quantities of either antifibrinolytic or progestogen have been shown to reduce menstrual blood loss.

d *F* Ethamsylate has not proven useful for the treatment of menorrhagia.

e *F* Mefenamic acid is taken during the time of the period.

24 a *T* Non-steroidal anti-inflammatory drugs have been shown to be effective in reducing dysmenorrhoea, reducing prostaglandin-induced uterine contractions.

b *F* Ovulatory menstrual cycles are typically associated with spasmodic dysmenorrhoea.

c *F* A retroverted uterus that is not associated with pelvic pathology is not responsible for an increased severity of dysmenorrhoea. (But a retroverted uterus that *is* associated with pelvic pathology *is* responsible for an increased severity of dysmenorrhoea.)

d *T* Dysmenorrhoea can be a prominent feature of women suffering from endometriosis.

e *F* Anterior vaginal wall prolapse is not associated with menstrually related discomfort or pain.

25 a *T* Taking the progesterone-only pill may be associated with either regular menstrual cycles, erratic vaginal bleeding or amenorrhoea.

b *T* The progesterone-only pill is safe to prescribe immediately following delivery.

c *F* There is no association between the progesterone-only pill and thromboembolic disease.

d *F* Only 40% of women taking the progesterone-only pill have their ovulation inhibited; the POP's main action is in thickening the cervical mucus, thus reducing sperm penetration.

e *F* The progesterone-only pill *decreases* tubal motility, hence its association with tubal ectopic pregnancy.

26 a *F* Expulsion of an intrauterine device is more common in nulliparous women compared with parous women. Expulsions vary between 1 and 10 per 100 women in the first year of use.

b *T* The addition of copper to the plastic frame increases contraceptive efficacy.

   c *T* Removal of an intrauterine contraceptive device in early pregnancy is warranted despite the risk of miscarriage, as the miscarriage risk is even greater if the device is left *in situ*.

   d *T* Past history of ectopic pregnancy is a relative contraindication.

   e *F* An intrauterine contraceptive device increases the risk of miscarriage, not fetal abnormality.

27 a *T* Epidurals causes venous 'pooling' and a fluid pre-load reduces the incidence of hypotension.

   b *T* The siting of an epidural is contraindicated in the presence of a coagulopathy because of the risk of bleeding from the venous sinuses and haematoma formation.

   c *T* An epidural causes peripheral dilation and pooling of the blood thereby lowering the maternal blood pressure.

   d *F* Epidurals are associated with an *increased* rate of forceps deliveries.

   e *T* A combined spinal epidural is helpful for elective deliveries, giving both acute and postnatal analgesia.

28 a *T* Amniotomy, which may need to be followed by an oxytocin infusion, is a successful means of inducing labour.

   b *F* The cervix is *least* favourable when in the posterior position. Anterior is best.

   c *F* Ergometrine causes tonic contraction of the uterus and is therefore inappropriate for the induction of labour.

   d *F* The highest chance of a successful vaginal delivery with a twin pregnancy is with the spontaneous onset of labour. Routine induction of labour cannot be justified at 36 weeks, but at 38 weeks is common practice.

   e *T* Intravenous prostaglandin infusion does cause uterine contractions but the unpleasant gastroenterological side effects mean it is not used in practice.

29 a *F* The first stage of labour requires the cervix to become fully dilated and is reliant upon adequate uterine activity. It is not restricted by the bony pelvis.

b *T* If inefficient uterine activity has been excluded, delay in the later part of the first stage of labour may be suggestive of cephalopelvic disproportion.

c *F* Maternal anaemia is not associated with delay in any stage of labour.

d *T* With the exception of the preterm fetus, a brow presentation is not normally deliverable vaginally and is an important presentation to exclude when delay in the first stage is noted.

e *T* Cessation of previously good progress in labour of a woman who has had a previous Caesarean section should alert the clinician to the possibility of scar tissue.

30 a *T* An episiotomy can overcome the problem of a rigid perineum delaying the second stage of labour.

b *F* The length of the umbilical cord varies greatly but in practice never prevents delivery.

c *F* The diagnosis of the second stage of labour cannot be made until full cervical dilatation has been achieved.

d *T* The lack of expulsive sensation in the presence of an adequately working epidural can cause the second stage to be prolonged.

e *T* Maternal exhaustion, which can be multifactorial, is a common cause of delay in the second stage.

Multiple-choice questions: Paper 2

1 Down's syndrome:
   a has a birth prevalence in the region of 1.4 per 1000 in England and Wales
   b can be diagnosed using serum screening
   c can be found in mosaic form
   d is associated with oligohydramnios
   e is associated with a higher rate of miscarriage than in pregnancies with a normal karyotype.

2 Concerning post-coital contraception.
   a The progesterone-only pill can be used.
   b Oral methods should be administered within 24 hours.
   c It is available as an 'over the counter' preparation.
   d The intrauterine device has a role.
   e Follow-up of individuals who have used post-coital contraception is not worthwhile.

3 Urinary tract infection in pregnancy:
   a is associated with preterm labour
   b is commonly due to staphylococci
   c acute pyelonephritis is associated with intrauterine growth retardation
   d is more common with a transverse lie
   e may present with vomiting.

4 Rubella in pregnancy:
  a means screening pregnant women by sampling for rubella antibodies is advised
  b is associated with recurrent miscarriage
  c is associated with the greatest incidence of congenital malformations when the infection occurs during the second trimester
  d is indicated by a rising titre of rubella-specific IgM levels following recent infection
  e is associated with a neural tube defect in the fetus.

5 Congenital abnormalities are associated with the following maternal infections:
  a hepatitis B
  b toxoplasmosis
  c cytomegalovirus
  d group B streptococcus
  e parvovirus.

6 Concerning thalassaemia in pregnancy.
  a Thalassaemia minor may be suspected on a blood film.
  b It most commonly occurs in women of African origin.
  c The carrier rate in the UK is approximately 1 in 10000.
  d A woman with β-thalassaemia minor can be reassured that the baby will be healthy.
  e Thalassaemia trait increases the likelihood of pre-eclampsia.

7 LHRH analogues:
  a can be used to treat endometriosis
  b rarely cause side effects
  c can be administered orally
  d are inexpensive preparations
  e act principally at the uterine level.

8 Concerning intermenstrual bleeding (IMB).

a IMB occurs in about 10% of normal menstrual cycles.

b Laparoscopy should be included as part of the investigation.

c A luteal phase progesterone is essential.

d IMB may be associated with ovulation.

e IMB is a feature of cervical intra-epithelial neoplasia.

9 Risks of combined oral contraceptive (COC) pill usage include:

a increased incidence of endometrial carcinoma

b pelvic inflammatory disease

c benign ovarian cysts

d hypotension

e increased risk of ovarian carcinoma.

10 Rotational delivery:

a may be preceded by a labour during which back pain is a prominent feature

b can be achieved using a silastic ventouse cup

c can be safely attempted when two-fifths of the fetal head is palpable per abdomen

d can correct a deep transverse arrest

e should be attempted with a fetal pH of 7.12.

11 In pregnancy, ultrasound:

a can diagnose fetal ascites

b anomaly scanning is usually carried out in the second trimester of pregnancy

c can establish fetal maturity at 34 weeks' gestation

d can diagnose a cleft lip

e is able to identify the fertilised ovum prior to implantation.

12 The following are known to be teratogenic:

a alcohol

b methyldopa

c warfarin

d aminoglycosides

e phenytoin.

13 Fallopian tube occlusion:
   a may be caused by chlamydial infection
   b is a common finding in pelvic endometriosis
   c when caused by infection most commonly ascends from the
      lower genital tract
   d may follow appendicitis
   e can be assessed using transvaginal ultrasound.

14 Gonorrhoea:
   a may cause blindness in the baby of an infected mother
   b is diagnosed by taking a high vaginal swab
   c may cause perihepatitis
   d may cause penile discharge
   e is caused by a Gram-positive diplococcus.

15 The following instructions are appropriate when advising on the
   use of the diaphragm.
   a Always use a spermicide.
   b Sterilise the diaphragm prior to insertion.
   c The diaphragm cannot be used at the same time as the sheath.
   d Refitting the diaphragm is required after childbirth.
   e The diaphragm must be left in place for at least six hours
      following intercourse.

16 Concerning sickle cell disorders in pregnancy.
   a Sickle cell disorders are most common in women of Asian
      origin.
   b A sickle cell crisis can be precipitated in conditions of
      heightened oxygen tension.
   c Sickle cell disorders are associated with an increased incidence
      of hypertension during pregnancy.
   d Sickle cell disease results from a variant on the alpha globin
      chain.
   e Partner screening is recommended during the second
      trimester.

17 Urodynamic investigations:
a are unnecessary in the patient who complains of stress incontinence
b can be conducted before excluding urinary infection
c cystometry measures the pressure/volume relationship of the bladder during filling and voiding
d could usefully include ultrasonography
e if normal, should show a bladder capacity of 250 mL.

18 The perinatal mortality rate:
a is usually expressed at the rate per thousand total births over one year
b is attributable to congenital malformations in 50% of cases
c in England and Wales is higher in those whose mother was born in Pakistan than in those whose mother was born in the West Indies
d falls with social class
e is lowest in mothers aged between 18 and 20 years.

19 Tocolysis to suppress preterm labour:
a ideally should be continued for 12 hours
b carries the risk of maternal pulmonary oedema if β-sympathomimetics are used
c is usually initiated with oral therapy
d may be employed beyond 34 weeks' gestation
e is exclusively a role for β-sympathomimetics.

20 Ovarian masses:
a are malignant in the presence of ascites
b include benign teratomas
c of germ cell origin may secrete hormones
d may be confused with developmental abnormalities of the renal tract
e if malignant can be reliably staged pre-operatively.

21 Concerning lactation.
   a Lactation is successfully suppressed by demand feeding to empty the engorged breasts.
   b Colostrum is secreted for seven days after the birth.
   c Bromocryptine promotes milk production.
   d Lactation will fall with Sheehan's syndrome.
   e The staphylococcus organism is associated with puerperal mastitis.

22 When massive post-partum haemorrhage occurs:
   a an anaesthetist is essential to assist in the management of the patient
   b initial cross-matching of three units of blood is sufficient
   c bimanual uterine compression has a role
   d uncross-matched O Rhesus-positive blood may be given in an emergency
   e bilateral uterine artery ligation may be necessary.

23 Secondary post-partum haemorrhage:
   a is abnormal bleeding that occurs 12 hours post-partum
   b may be due to infection
   c cannot be controlled by uterine contracting agents
   d occurs following 5% of births
   e can usually be diagnosed by ultrasound examination of the pelvic organs.

24 Regarding resuscitation of the newborn.
   a Resuscitation in some form is required in approximately one-third of babies.
   b The Apgar score is recorded at delivery.
   c Resuscitation will be required if the fetal heart rate is persistently 90 beats a minute.
   d Meconium seen in the posterior pharynx and larynx is an indication for intubation.
   e Naloxone can be given safely to all infants.

25 Concerning maternal cardiac disease in pregnancy.
  a A classification system exists to determine the mortality risk.
  b Involvement of the aorta in Marfan's syndrome increases the mortality.
  c The fetus has an increased risk of congenital heart disease.
  d Mitral stenosis is an infrequent complication following rheumatic heart disease.
  e Women with primary pulmonary hypertension should be advised against pregnancy.

26 Appropriate maternal investigations following a term stillbirth would include:
  a glycosylated haemoglobin
  b a Kleihauer blood test
  c a platelet count
  d blood pressure measurement
  e antinuclear antibody estimation.

27 Placental abruption:
  a may have no associated vaginal bleeding
  b is an indication for delivery
  c has a higher incidence with maternal cocaine abuse
  d may be identified using ultrasound to demonstrate retroplacental clot
  e can be readily distinguished from acute appendicitis.

28 The ventouse method:
  a may employ a metal cup
  b has increased in popularity with electronic pumps
  c can be used safely in the absence of criteria necessary for a forceps delivery
  d requires the patient to be in the lithotomy position
  e may be performed in conjunction with a pudendal block.

29 A high fetal head at term in a primipara:
  a can be caused by placenta praevia
  b can be caused by a lower-segment uterine fibroid

c is associated with incorrect pregnancy dating

d is an indication for a Caesarean section

e has a higher incidence in patients of African origin.

30 Fetal well-being in the third trimester can be usefully assessed by:

a serial assessment of symphyseal fundal height

b ultrasound measurement of crown–rump length

c ultrasound measurement of amniotic fluid volume

d measuring serum alpha-fetoprotein

e measuring serum oestradiol levels.

Answers: MCQs Paper 2

1 a *T* This figure translates into approximately 970 affected births annually.

   b *F* The serum screening only gives a risk for the likely incidence of Down's syndrome being present at term in an individual pregnancy. Diagnosis requires karyotyping.

   c *T* Mosaicism accounts for 1–2% of Down's cases.

   d *F* Polyhydramnios is found in association with duodenal atresia.

   e *T* Fetal wastage is more common with all types of chromosomal abnormalities.

2 a *F* The POP is not used in this context, as its principal mechanism of action is thickening of cervical mucus and prevention of sperm penetration.

   b *F* It should be administered within 72 hours.

   c *T* Post-coital contraception is available for purchase over the counter.

   d *T* Following adequate counselling the intrauterine contraceptive device may be fitted within five days of the episode of unprotected intercourse.

   e *F* Follow-up can detect method failures and ensure adequate contraceptive measures are being taken.

3 a *T* Uterine activity can be precipitated by urinary infection and should always be screened for and treated in the patient who presents with symptoms and/or signs of preterm labour.

   b *F* This organism is unusual; the most common bacterium found is *Escherichia coli*.

   c *T* This association, together with the risks of preterm labour and delivery, is the indication for hospitalisation and intravenous antibiotic therapy to treat acute pyelonephritis.

   d *F* There is no known, statistically proven association with fetal lie.

   e *T* A variety of non-specific symptoms may be present, such as nausea, vomiting, fever and abdominal pain.

4 a *T* Such screening provides valuable baseline information. Additionally, all women who lack rubella antibodies should be identified and offered postnatal vaccination.

  b *F* A pregnancy during which primary rubella infection is contracted has a higher incidence of miscarriage. Thereafter rubella immunity is developed and protects a subsequent pregnancy from this complication.

  c *F* First-trimester infection has the most devastating consequences, with in excess of 80% of fetuses affected.

  d *T* Detection of rising IgM titres is used for diagnostic purposes. Rubella-specific IgM is demonstrable for up to eight weeks after the onset of the rash.

  e *F* A variety of defects, including cataracts, chorioretinitis, microphthalmia, glaucoma, deafness, microcephaly and mental retardation but not neural tube defects, are associated with congenital rubella infection.

5 a *F* There is no known association. However, infants born to hepatitis B surface-antigen-positive women should be given hepatitis B immunoglobulin and active immunisation shortly after delivery.

  b *T* Toxoplasmosis infection is associated with fetal intracranial calcification, microcephaly, hydrocephaly and hepatosplenomegaly.

  c *T* Cytomegalovirus can result in hepatosplenomegaly, microcephaly, hyperbilirubinaemia, petechiae and thrombocytopenia.

  d *F* Group B streptococcus is a common normal maternal vaginal commensal. It does not cause fetal abnormality. It can cause overwhelming neonatal infections, but this is rare.

  e *F* Parvovirus B19 infection is a known cause of non-immune hydrops fetalis. This is not a congenital abnormality.

6 a *T* Red blood cells of sufferers are small, with a low mean cell volume and low mean cell haemoglobin.

  b *F* Thalassaemia has a worldwide distribution but is concentrated in a broad band encompassing the Mediterranean and Middle East.

    c *T* The carrier rate of approximately 1 in 10 000 in the UK can be compared with a carrier rate of 1 in 7 in Cyprus.

    d *F* Depending on the carrier status of the mother's partner, the fetus may have a normal haemoglobin, thalassaemia minor or thalassaemia major. Therefore, no such reassurance can be given.

    e *F* There is no known association.

7 a *T* LHRH analogues have proved to be successful therapy for endometriosis in a number of controlled trials.

    b *F* Side effects similar to those experienced by women during the menopause are commonly experienced by women in receipt of LHRH analogue treatment.

    c *F* The polypeptide structure of the LHRH analogues makes them inappropriate for oral administration. Parenteral routes, including the nasal route, injection and depot preparations, have been developed.

    d *F* Costs of these preparations are in excess of £80 per month.

    e *F* LHRH analogues act by initial stimulation, followed by down-regulation of pituitary gonadotrophin secretion.

8 a *F* IMB is uncommon in the normal menstrual cycle.

    b *F* *Hysteroscopy* is the more useful investigation.

    c *F* The establishment of ovulation is not essential in the management of patients with IMB, but it may be helpful if progestogens are to be considered in the adequately assessed anovulatory patient.

    d *T* Regular mid-cycle spotting and pain ('mittelschmerz') are noted by some women at the time of ovulation.

    e *F* Pre-invasive cervical disease does not cause IMB.

9 a *F* The COC has a protective effect in the order of 50%.

    b *F* The incidence of PID is *lower* in women who use the COC as a method of contraception, compared with women who have unprotected intercourse.

    c *F* The incidence of benign ovarian cysts is *lower*.

    d *F* COC usage is associated with *hypertension*.

    e *F* The COC has a protective effect; most studies indicate a reduction in excess of 50%.

10 a *T* Back pain is common in labours with an occipito-posterior position of the fetal head.

b *T* The ventouse has increased in popularity for achieving safe rotational vaginal delivery. Clinicians often prefer the metal cup for rotations, feeling the failure rate is lower.

c *F* None of the head should be palpable per abdomen.

d *T* Rotation to the occipito-anterior position can permit vaginal delivery.

e *F* In the presence of fetal distress, delivery should be by Caesarean section.

11 a *T* Fluid can clearly be seen around the fetal liver and bowel.

b *T* Most commonly this examination is now conducted around 20 weeks of gestational age

c *F* Fetal maturity cannot be reliably determined ultrasonographically in the third trimester.

d *T* Early diagnosis of cleft lip can be useful information to forewarn the parents and paediatric surgeons.

e *F* Pregnancies can only be detected following implantation.

12 a *T* Widespread abnormalities, including those of the fetal alcohol syndrome with growth retardation, central nervous system abnormalities, microcephaly, microphthalmia and poorly developed philtrum, have been described.

b *F* Methyldopa has been used safely during pregnancy for many years to control hypertension. There have been occasional case reports of microcephaly.

c *T* Warfarin is known to cause intracerebral haemorrhage, nasal hypoplasia and stippling of the epiphyses.

d *T* Aminoglycosides are known to be ototoxic.

e *T* Phenytoin can cause fetal hydantoin syndrome. Various craniofacial and digital abnormalities, together with more major anomalies (cardiac defects, cleft lip and palate), have been associated with maternal phenytoin ingestion during pregnancy.

13 a *T* Chlamydial infection, which may be asymptomatic, can cause considerable tubal damage. It is more common than gonorrhoea as the infection responsible.

b *F* Tubal occlusion is surprisingly uncommon even in the presence of moderately severe pelvic endometriosis.

c *T* The mechanism, however, by which infection ascends through the cervical canal and reaches the fallopian tubes is still unknown.

d *T* Appendicitis can result in tubal damage, both from the local pelvic inflammatory reaction and the associated surgery.

e *F* A hydrosalpinx may be seen ultrasonographically, but occlusion of normal calibre tube and fimbrial end clubbing cannot be diagnosed by this means.

14 a *T* Gonococcal ophthalmia neonatorum can lead to severe conjunctivitis, keratitis and blindness if not promptly treated.

b *F* Endocervical and urethral swabs are required. In some circumstances throat and rectal swabs should be considered.

c *T* Systemic manifestations, perihepatitis and septicaemia can all be caused by gonococcal infection.

d *T* The majority of gonococcal-infected men develop a urethritis, dysuria and urethral discharge.

e *F* Gonococcus is a Gram-*negative* intracellular diplococcus.

15 a *T* The efficacy of the diaphragm as a method of contraception is reduced if this advice is ignored.

b *F* The diaphragm should be clean, but sterility is not required.

c *F* Safer sexual practices are to be encouraged and there is no reason why two barrier methods should not be used together.

d *T* It is important to advise refitting after each child is born and when there has been a significant weight change in the user.

e *T* Removal before six hours has elapsed following intercourse diminishes the efficacy of the diaphragm method of contraception. If further intercourse takes place before this time, the spermicide should be replenished.

16 a *F* African and West Indian populations have the highest incidence.

b *F* *Lowered* oxygen tension, acidosis, infection and dehydration may precipitate a crisis.

c *T* Regular screening for hypertension/pre-eclampsia, urinary tract infection and reduced fetal growth is recommended in women with sickle cell disease.

d *F* Sickle cell disease results from an amino acid substitution of glutamine for valine on the *beta* globin chain.

e *F* Earlier (pre-pregnancy or first trimester) diagnosis is recommended so that the couple can be advised on the possible risk of a serious haemoglobin defect in their offspring and subsequently counselled about prenatal diagnostic options.

17 a *F* Studies have shown that a significant proportion of women with stress incontinence have detrusor instability and therefore this investigation is worthwhile to prevent inappropriate intervention.

b *F* Urinary infection may be responsible for some or even all of a patient's symptoms and therefore if should always be excluded before conducting time-consuming and invasive investigations.

c *T* Cystometry is indicated in the investigation of patients with multiple symptoms, a voiding disorder, previous unsuccessful incontinence surgery or a neuropathic bladder disorder.

d *T* Ultrasound is a means of assessing post-micturition residual urinary volume and the bladder neck.

e *F* Capacity (taken as a strong desire to void) should be greater than 400 mL.

18 a *T* The perinatal mortality rate is the number of perinatal deaths divided by the total births (born live and still) expressed as a proportion of 1000 total births occurring in the same location during the same period.

b *F* *Twenty per cent* of deaths are attributable to congenital malformations.

c *T* Mothers from Pakistan also have a higher perinatal mortality rate than those from India and Bangladesh.

d *F* Perinatal mortality *rises* with social class.

e *F* Perinatal mortality is lowest in those mothers aged between 20 and 29 years.

19 a *F* Labour should be suppressed for *24–48* hours to gain maximum benefit from the steroids used to enhance fetal lung development.

b *T* Maternal pulmonary oedema is a particular risk with the β-sympathomimetics and warrants careful attention to the patient's fluid balance.

c *F* Intravenous therapy is almost universally administered initially, the role of oral tocolysis remaining controversial.

d *T* Although permitting delivery is the usual management when gestation has reached 34 weeks, tocolysis may temporarily suppress labour, enabling *in utero* transfer to a unit with more sophisticated obstetric and neonatal facilities.

e *F* Atosiban, magnesium sulphate, indomethacin and nifedipine are some of the alternative pharmacological agents that have been investigated.

20 a *F* Ascites can occur with benign ovarian tumours and parasitic fibroids. Meig's syndrome describes ascites and pleural effusion in association with a benign ovarian fibroma.

b *T* Teratomas (also known as dermoids) are most common in young women and are bilateral in about 12% of cases.

c *T* Both α-fetoprotein and human chorionic gonadotrophin may be produced.

d *T* A palpable pelvic kidney can simulate an ovarian mass.

e *F* Careful surgical staging is essential to determine the appropriate subsequent management.

21 a *F* Such measures *promote* milk production. Non-feeding, simple analgesia and a good supportive bra are usually adequate measures.

b *F* Colostrum is secreted for approximately the first two days post-partum; the change to milk occurs on the third and fourth day.

c *F* Bromocryptine inhibits the release of prolactin from the pituitary and is therefore useful for the suppression of lactation.

d *T* Sheehan's syndrome or necrosis of the anterior pituitary following severe post-partum haemorrhage is now fortunately very rare. If the patient survives, there is a failure of lactation due to the lack of prolactin and manifestations of the other endocrine deficiencies.

e *T* Mastitis is associated with milk stasis, nipple trauma and poor nursing technique. Pathogenic bacteria enter and are most commonly of the staphylococcal type.

22 a *T* The anaesthetist is an essential member of the team and will normally manage the patient's fluid balance, in addition to inserting central intravenous access lines.

b *F* A minimum of six units of blood should be cross-matched.

c *T* Uterine atony resulting in dramatic bleeding may be controlled by forcibly compressing the uterus between a hand on the abdomen and a hand inserted *per vaginum*.

d *F* Uncross-matched O Rhesus-*negative* blood can be used unless the patient is known to have blood group antibodies.

e *T* Uterine haemorrhage that cannot be controlled by local or pharmacological means necessitates surgery. Uterine artery ligation may be sufficient to avoid hysterectomy.

23 a *F* Secondary post-partum haemorrhage is defined as abnormal bleeding that occurs between 24 hours and six weeks post-partum.

b *T* Infection is a common cause.

c *F* Uterine relaxation and atony can occur in the few days following delivery. It may respond to oxytocin, ergometrine or prostaglandin therapy. The possibility of retained products, however, should be borne in mind.

d *F* Secondary post-partum haemorrhage occurs after *1*% of births.

e *F* Ultrasonically, it may be difficult to distinguish retained products from blood clot and it may not be diagnostic.

24 a *T* Although some form of resuscitation is required in about a third of babies, active resuscitation, such as assisted ventilation, is required by less than 5%.

    b *F* The Apgar score is recorded at 1, 5 and sometimes 10 minutes after delivery.

    c *T* Recognition of the need for resuscitation should be prompt (in the first minute) if there is no regular respiration, if the heart rate is below 100 beats/minute or if the Apgar score remains below 7.

    d *T* Gentle suction should be applied to the endotracheal tube until no further meconium is obtained, changing the tube should it become blocked during the process.

    e *F* Care should be taken in the infant of a mother who is a known opiate addict. Use may precipitate acute withdrawal in the neonate.

25 a *T* The New York Heart Association Classification is based on the physical abilities of the mother and is divided into four classes. Nearly 90% are in the milder categories of 1 and 2; those with class 3 and 4 account for only 10% of heart disease in pregnancy but account for 85% of cardiac-caused deaths.

    b *T* Involvement of the aorta in Marfan's syndrome increases the mortality from 5–15% to 25–50%.

    c *T* The fetus has a greater risk of congenital heart disease when the abnormality is present on the maternal side rather than the paternal one. There is also an increased incidence of prematurity and intrauterine growth retardation.

    d *F* Mitral stenosis is the more frequent rheumatic valvular disorder (90%).

    e *T* Primary pulmonary hypertension is associated with sudden death; the raised cardiac output and decreased peripheral resistance of normal pregnancy increases the risk to an unacceptable 50%.

26 a *T* Maternal glycosylated haemoglobin is required for the detection of diabetes mellitus, as glycaemia control may have returned to within normal limits post-partum.

　 b *T* A Kleihauer blood test is an acid-stained film of maternal blood to establish the presence of fetal red blood cells and quantitate the volume of feto-maternal transfusion.

　 c *T* An increasing incidence of consumptive coagulopathy develops with time following fetal demise and therefore should be checked in a woman with a retained dead fetus *in utero*.

　 d *T* Hypertensive disease of all aetiologies increases perinatal mortality.

　 e *T* Systemic lupus erythematosus is associated with an increased pregnancy loss in all trimesters.

27 a *T* So-called 'concealed' abruptions constitute 20–35% of cases.

　 b *F* In cases of mild abruption, particularly with the preterm fetus, provided the fetal condition is monitored, expectant management should be considered.

　 c *T* Maternal cocaine abuse is associated with a higher incidence of placental abruption and increased risks of growth retardation and preterm labour.

　 d *T* The diagnosis of placental abruption is principally a clinical one, but in the presence of a large clot it may be identified as a hyperechogenic area on ultrasound examination.

　 e *F* The diagnosis of appendicitis in pregnancy is notoriously difficult and can be confused with concealed placental abruption.

28 a *T* Pliable silastic cups are increasing in popularity and replacing the metal cups, as they are simpler to assemble.

　 b *T* Electronic pumps produce a rapid onset and reliably controlled vacuum and are therefore preferred to the hand-pump devices.

　 c *F* The criteria for the ventouse method and forceps should be the same.

　 d *T* The patient should be in the lithotomy position, similar to a forceps delivery.

e *T* A pudendal block may be adequate with perineal infiltration of local anaesthetic for the lift-out procedures.

29 a *T* A placenta which significantly encroaches into the lower segment prevents engagement of the fetal head.

b *T* Any 'tumour' which obstructs the lower segment can prevent descent of the fetal head.

c *T* The preterm infant would not be expected to have engaged in the pelvis and therefore the dating of the pregnancy should be checked. The widespread use of early ultrasound has assisted in the more accurate assessment of pregnancy gestation.

d *F* Significant numbers will experience descent of the head into the pelvis during labour and successful vaginal delivery and therefore routine Caesarean section cannot be justified. The possibility of cephalopelvic disproportion should, however, be borne in mind.

e *T* African races commonly have a pelvic inlet with a higher angle of inclination than Caucasian women and therefore the head may fail to engage before the onset of labour.

30 a *T* Serial assessments of symphysial fundal height are useful at picking up growth restriction, although ideally these measurements should be done by the same person.

b *F* Crown–rump length is used in the first trimester.

c *T* Reduced amniotic fluid is associated with impaired fetal renal function.

d *F* Serum alpha-fetoprotein levels are not useful in the third trimester.

e *F* Oestriol levels have been used in the past but oestradiol levels are unhelpful.

Multiple-choice questions: Paper 3

3

1 Concerning infections of the genital tract.
   a Vaginal candidiasis predisposes to oral infections of the neonate.
   b *Gardnerella vaginalis* is encouraged by an increase in the number of Döderleins bacilli in the vagina.
   c Vaginal discharge due to *Candida albicans* is effectively treated by metronidazole.
   d Metronidazole is contraindicated in pregnancy.
   e Gonorrhoea causes bartholinitis.

2 Cervical polyps:
   a cause spontaneous abortion
   b are a cause of ante-partum haemorrhage
   c cause watery vaginal discharge
   d are covered by squamous epithelium
   e cause intermenstrual bleeding.

3 Regarding female micturition.
   a Retention of urine may be due to an enterocele.
   b Urge incontinence associated with detrusor instability is improved by pelvic floor exercises.
   c Detrusor instability is associated with upper motor neurone lesions.
   d If a woman presents with mainly stress incontinence, urodynamics are not needed.
   e Acute retention may be due to haematocolpos.

4 Prolapse:
  a may prevent complete emptying of the bladder
  b is more common in women of African origin
  c if second degree may be treated by a Hodge pessary
  d is associated with vaginal bleeding
  e occurs only after the menopause.

5 Transverse lie:
  a is associated with a double uterus
  b is associated with multiple pregnancy
  c is the commonest lie of the second twin
  d can be found with an ante-partum haemorrhage
  e should be delivered by classical Caesarean section.

6 Regarding the maternal mortality report for the years 2003–5.
  a Substandard care was implicated in nearly 25% of deaths.
  b The main causes of direct maternal deaths were hypertensive disorders and cerebral haemorrhage.
  c The number of maternal deaths due to haemorrhage had increased since the previous triennium.
  d Deaths due to anaesthesia had decreased.
  e About 25% of the women who died from direct or indirect causes were either overweight or obese.

7 Regarding carcinoma of the endometrium.
  a Risk factors include opposed HRT.
  b It can be diagnosed by an endometrial biopsy.
  c Common UK treatment is a radical hysterectomy followed by external beam radiotherapy.
  d The incidence is lower in thin women, as they have more conversion of androgen precursors to oestrone.
  e It can be preceded by cystic or adenomatous hyperplasia.

8 Regarding uterine inversion.
  a It should not occur if the third stage of labour is managed appropriately.

   b It should prompt suspicion of morbid adherence of the placenta.

   c If the placenta is attached, it should be removed immediately.

   d It can be replaced by the hydrostatic method.

   e The uterus should not be replaced before anaesthesia (GA, epidural or spinal) is administered.

9   Concerning the vulva.

   a Unilateral enlargement can be due to a hydrocele of the canal of Gordon.

   b Pruritis vulvae can be caused by pox virus.

   c With atrophic dystrophies testosterone cream may be useful.

   d Vulval carcinoma forms about 10% of all female genital tract cancers.

   e Vulval carcinoma may present with the symptoms of intractable pruritis.

10 A woman presents with a history of seven weeks' amenorrhoea followed by six weeks of mild vaginal bleeding.

   a She may have a tubal pregnancy.

   b If the serum beta HCG is < 5 an ectopic is excluded.

   c She may be miscarrying.

   d She may have retained products of conception.

   e If she has dysfunctional uterine bleeding high-dose progestogens should stop the bleeding.

11 Regarding neonatal medicine.

   a All normal-term babies lose weight after delivery but regain their birthweight by five days.

   b Neonates with phenylketonuria should not be breastfed.

   c Erythema toxicum has a high mortality.

   d Jaundice occurring in the first 24 hours is most likely to be physiological and is due to increased unconjugated bilirubin levels.

   e Excessive oxygen administration in the preterm infant can cause retinopathy.

12 Regarding male fertility.
  a Azoospermia may respond to steroid treatment.
  b In a semen sample five white blood cells (WBCs) per high-power field is normal.
  c In a semen sample 40% of abnormal forms is acceptable.
  d Low FSH and LH suggest testicular failure.
  e Micromanipulation of the zona pellucida increases fertility rates.

13 Laparoscopies:
  a have a mortality rate of approximately 1 in 30000
  b may be complicated by an H_2O embolus
  c commonly produce shoulder-tip pain postoperatively
  d should always be preceded by emptying of the bladder
  e can cause peritonitis.

14 Regarding hydatidiform mole.
  a The incidence is higher in Indonesia than in Australia.
  b The uterus may be smaller than the dates signify.
  c It may present with symptoms and signs of pre-eclampsia.
  d It must be followed up by the local hospital.
  e A subsequent pregnancy can stimulate a recurrence.

15 A woman suddenly collapses five minutes after a normal delivery.
  a The first priorities are to insert an IV line, then establish an airway, then ventilate.
  b If she has had an amniotic fluid embolism, she may develop disseminated intravascular coagulopathy (DIC).
  c If she is likely having a massive post-partum haemorrhage, the most likely cause is a cervical tear.
  d She has had a previous Caesarean section, but as she has just had a normal delivery, uterine rupture could not be a cause.
  e A pulmonary embolus is unlikely as she has had a normal delivery.

16 The following conditions cause ambiguous external genitalia in the neonate:
  a Turner's syndrome
  b testicular feminisation (androgen insensitivity)

c cryptorchidism

d adrenogenital syndrome

e Klinefelter's syndrome.

17 The following changes occur in the mother during normal pregnancy.
   a The blood urea level falls to 3.0 mmol/L or less.
   b There is a decrease in mucoid discharge from the cervix.
   c Respiratory tidal volume falls.
   d There is an increase in cardiac output by eight weeks' gestation.
   e Fasting blood glucose levels in the first trimester are greater than in the non-pregnant state.

18 In severe pre-eclampsia:
   a the creatinine clearance rate is higher than in normal pregnancy
   b there are defects of the development of the placental bed in the second trimester
   c there is an increased incidence of placental abruption
   d the intravascular compartment is increased
   e plasma urea levels are raised.

19 Regarding Rhesus disease.
   a Anti-D should be given if antibodies are detected in early pregnancy.
   b It may be caused by genetic amniocentesis.
   c Rhesus disease is routinely prevented by giving anti-D gammaglobulin in the first trimester of pregnancy.
   d There is no increased risk if the Kleihauer test is negative.
   e It is more likely to occur in a Rhesus-negative mother with an ABO-incompatible fetus.

20 The fetal head is said to be engaged when:
   a it becomes fixed in the pelvic brim
   b the leading part is 1 cm above the ischial spines
   c the biparietal diameter has passed through the pelvic brim
   d one-fifth of the fetal head is palpable abdominally
   e the caput succedaneum reaches the level of the ischial spines.

21 Ovulation in the human:
   a   is accompanied by a surge of follicle-stimulating hormone
   b   is characteristically followed by the development of secretory endometrium
   c   is followed by increased ferning of the cervical mucus
   d   is associated with a sustained rise in basal body temperature
   e   occurs 14 days before the next menstrual period.

22 Regarding HRT in the postmenopausal woman.
   a   With a history of thromboembolic disease, oral therapy is preferable to transdermal.
   b   Premarin 0.625 mg is adequate for prevention of bone loss.
   c   Cystic hyperplasia must be treated by Wertheim's hysterectomy.
   d   An endometrial thickness of 3 mm suggests hyperplasia if she is taking continuous combined therapy.
   e   Oestrogen replacement therapy will decrease HDL levels.

23 In vaginal breech delivery:
   a   delay in the second stage is usually treated by oxytocin
   b   it is best managed by extraction soon after full cervical dilatation
   c   when the legs are extended the presenting diameter is the ditrochanteric
   d   the commonest cause of perinatal death is prematurity
   e   the fetal back (sacrum) should be kept posterior.

24 Regarding maternal mortality in the UK.
   a   The maternal mortality rate during 2003–5 was 14 per 10 000 births.
   b   Deaths related to hypertension are most commonly caused by cardiac failure.
   c   Emergency general anaesthesia contributes to death from Mendelssohn's syndrome.
   d   Cardiac disease was the most common cause of indirect death.
   e   In modern obstetrics amniotic fluid embolism should be preventable.

25 Hyperprolactinaemia:
  a is a cause of infertility in women
  b may be treated with dopamine antagonist drugs
  c may be difficult to diagnose with certainty
  d can by physiological
  e is caused by an adenoma of the posterior pituitary gland.

26 The premenstrual syndrome (PMS):
  a has a low placebo response rate
  b may respond to dietary manipulation
  c diagnosis must be supported by written or visual evidence
  d can be treated by ovulation suppression
  e does not respond to mefenamic acid.

27 Regarding syphilis.
  a Palmar rash is a sign of secondary syphilis.
  b The primary chancre heals spontaneously after five to eight days.
  c Presenting signs are often condylomata acuminata.
  d The regional lymph nodes become enlarged, soft and very tender in primary disease.
  e Secondary syphilis has a low infectivity.

28 Carcinoma of the cervix:
  a classically presents with post-coital, intermenstrual or postmenopausal bleeding
  b if stage 1b, it can be treated with a Wertheim's hysterectomy and conservation of the ovaries
  c if treated surgically is usually followed with chemotherapy
  d has had a decreased incidence since introduction of the cervical screening programme in the UK
  e can present with urinary incontinence.

29 Polycystic ovarian syndrome:
  a is also known as Stein-Curtis syndrome
  b may be treated with clomiphene
  c may present with alopecia
  d is associated with raised LH and FSH levels
  e commonly presents with menorrhagia.

30 Regarding partograms.

  a The slowest acceptable rate of progress in a multiparous woman is 1 cm every two hours.

  b If delay occurs in the second stage in a primigravida, oxytocin must not be used.

  c If delay occurs at 7 cm in a multiparous woman, inefficient uterine action is the commonest cause.

  d They are graphic descriptions of labour.

  e They are only useful if vaginal examinations are documented every two hours.

Answers: MCQs Paper 3

1 a *T* Vaginal candidiasis can be transmitted to the fetus at the time of vaginal delivery.

    b *F* *Gardnerella vaginalis* is *discouraged* by an increase in the number of Döderleins bacilli in the vagina, as the latter act to lower the pH of the vagina.

    c *F* Vaginal candidiasis is treated by local therapy, e.g. clotrimazole pessaries or oral therapy, e.g. fluconazole.

    d *F* Metronidazole can be given throughout pregnancy but, as with all drugs, is best avoided in the first trimester.

    e *T* Gonorrhoea can cause bartholinitis, cervicitis, urethritis, pelvic disease and inflammatory disease.

2 a *F* Cervical polyps do not cause miscarriage.

    b *T* Cervical polyps can cause bleeding at any time either in the non-pregnant or pregnant state. The majority, however, are asymptomatic.

    c *F* Watery discharge is usually due to infection or very rarely to tubal carcinoma; it would be a most unusual presentation for a cervical polyp.

    d *F* Cervical polyps are covered by columnar epithelium.

    e *T* Cervical polyps can cause both intermenstrual and post-coital bleeding.

3 a *F* An enterocele is a prolapse of the pouch of Douglas which may contain bowel or omentum and does not affect bladder function.

    b *F* Pelvic floor exercises may improve stress incontinence. Bladder drill is more useful in the patient with detrusor instability.

    c *T* Upper motor neurone lesions are associated with a hyper-reflexic or so-called 'neuropathic' bladder.

    d *F* Urodynamics should be performed in all women with incontinence. Symptoms of stress incontinence may be caused by detrusor contractions.

    e *T* Any mass in the pelvis can cause acute urinary retention, including retained blood in the vagina secondary to an imperforate hymen.

4 a *T* If there is a large cystocele and significant uterine prolapse, there may be persistent residual urine in the bladder following voiding.

   b *F* African women rarely suffer utero-vaginal prolapse, the reason for this remaining uncertain.

   c *F* A Hodge pessary is used for anteversion of a retroverted uterus. A ring or shelf pessary may be used for uterine prolapse.

   d *T* A procidentia can become ulcerated and cause bleeding.

   e *F* The factor contributing most to utero-vaginal prolapse is childbirth, so premenopausal women can have this problem, although the condition may deteriorate when the tissues become oestrogen deficient with ovarian failure.

5 a *F* A 'double' (didelphic) uterus acts as a single uterus. It is the more subtle Müllerian duct abnormalities (e.g. arcuate uterus) that result in abnormal presentations.

   b *T* Multiple pregnancies have a higher incidence of transverse lie and all other malpresentations.

   c *F* The commonest presentation of a second twin is cephalic, followed by a breech.

   d *T* If the placenta is in the lower segment or overlying the cervix, i.e. placenta praevia, there will be an increased chance of a transverse lie.

   e *F* In the presence of ruptured membranes and a preterm fetus a classical Caesarean section may be necessary but each case must be considered individually. At term the transverse fetus is usually delivered at Caesarean section by bringing the legs down and out of the wound first.

6 a *F* Substandard care was evident in nearly 50% of the reported cases of direct and indirect deaths.

   b *F* The main causes of direct maternal deaths were thrombosis and thromboembolism, hypertensive disorders and haemorrhage.

   c *F* The number due to haemorrhage has slightly decreased since the last triennium.

   d *F* Deaths due to anaesthesia have remained the same.

e *F* More than half were either overweight or obese and 15% were morbidly or super morbidly obese.

7 a *F* If oestrogen replacement therapy is given in conjunction with 12 days of progestogen therapy, the incidence of carcinoma of the endometrium is decreased.

b *T* An endometrial biopsy will provide a histological diagnosis.

c *F* Treatment is usually a total abdominal hysterectomy with bilateral salpingo-oophorectomy and may be followed by radiotherapy, depending on the depth of endometrial involvement.

d *T* Obese women have more conversion of androgen precursors to oestrone and so have a higher incidence.

e *T* Endometrial hyperplasia without atypia carries a small risk (around 25%) of developing malignancy, but the presence of atypical cells increases the risk.

8 a *T* Correct management of the third stage involves placing a hand suprapubically to prevent inversion of the uterus when the placenta is delivered. However, the aetiology in some women remains uncertain.

b *T* Placenta accreta or percreta must be considered in the presence of uterine inversion.

c *F* Removal of an attached placenta in this situation may cause uncontrollable bleeding.

d *T* If initial manual attempts at replacing the uterus have failed, then the hydrostatic method is used.

e *F* Replacement should be attempted as soon as uterine inversion occurs by placing a fist beneath the inverted fundus and pushing cephalad. If this procedure is delayed, then the oedema of the tissues occurs, making replacement even more difficult.

9 a *F* Unilateral enlargement can be due to a hydrocoele of the canal of *Nuck*.

b *T* Pox virus (*Molluscum contagiosum*), as with other viral infections (herpes, warts), can cause itchy vulva.

c *T* Testosterone cream (2%) may be of value in atrophic vulval lesions. Commonly aqueous cream or hydrocortisone ointments are tried initially.

d *F* Vulval carcinoma forms about 5% of all genital tract cancers.

e *T* Because of this rather embarrassing complaint, presentation is often delayed. Physicians should also not hesitate to inspect the vulva prior to prescribing topical therapy.

10 a *T* Chronic ectopic pregnancies can present in this way.

b *T* An undetectable serum beta HCG will exclude an ectopic pregnancy

c *T* An incomplete miscarriage may present with a history of this nature. The diagnosis is often made by ultrasound if the clinical findings are not conclusive.

d *T* Retained products of conception can cause prolonged bleeding and are associated with risk of infection.

e *T* Prolonged bleeding due to hormonal causes will usually respond to high-dose progestogens. Alternatively oestrogens can be tried.

11 a *F* All normal-term babies will lose up to 10% of their birthweight in the first few days of life; however, birthweight should be regained by *7–10* days.

b *T* Babies with inborn errors of metabolism should not be breastfed, as they require specifically artificially manipulated feeds.

c *F* Erythema toxicum (urticaria neonatorum) occurs in the first week of life and is of uncertain cause but harmless.

d *F* Physiological jaundice commences on days two to four of life and is due to increased unconjugated bilirubin levels. Onset of jaundice in the first 24 hours of life is abnormal and requires investigation.

e *T* Oxygen administration in preterm infants can cause retrolental fibroplasia and in severe cases can lead to blindness.

12 a *F* There is no treatment for azoospermia unless it is due to a vasectomy, in which case re-anastomosis of the vas deferens may be successful.

b *F* No WBCs are normally seen in a semen sample.

c *T* A maximum of up to 50% of abnormal forms is acceptable in a semen sample.

d *F* Testicular failure produces *high* FSH and LH levels.

e *T* Micromanipulation allows easier entry of the spermatozoon into the zygote. Its usefulness has been proven in cases of poorly motile sperm.

13 a *F* Laparoscopies have a mortality of approximately 1 in 15 000, although this may vary with the increasing use of laparoscopic surgery.

b *F* CO$_2$ embolus is a complication which can occur in laparoscopy. This gas is used to insufflate the abdomen through a Veress needle.

c *T* CO$_2$ left in the abdominal cavity can irritate the diaphragm postoperatively and cause shoulder-tip pain via the phrenic nerve.

d *T* The bladder must be empty before insertion of the Veress needle.

e *T* Peritoneal infection can result from laparoscopies by direct introduction of bacteria, by damaging internal organs or by injecting dye through the cervix into the upper genital tract.

14 a *T* The large differences in various populations may have been exaggerated by selection bias. In the US and England rates of incidence between 0.5 and 2 per 1000 pregnancies have been reported.

b *T* The uterus may be larger, equivalent or smaller than expected for the expected gestation.

c *T* Vaginal bleeding is the most common presenting symptom. Theca lutein ovarian cysts are not infrequent and their presence is associated with hyperemesis and pre-eclampsia.

d *F* Regional centres (Charing Cross Hospital in London) operate a computerised follow-up system. Patients are contacted directly and urine or serum samples for β-HCG sent through the post.

e   *T*   Following any subsequent pregnancy HCG levels should be estimated to ensure that they have fallen to insignificant levels.

15   a   *F*   As with all cases of collapse the priorities are Airway, Breathing and Circulation.

    b   *T*   As thromboplastin is released into the circulation, DIC rapidly develops and may be impossible to correct.

    c   *F*   The most likely cause is an atonic uterus; a cervical tear is rare. A systematic approach to the patient ensures that all possibilities are investigated.

    d   *F*   A uterine dehiscence should always be thought of in women with a previous Caesarean section.

    e   *F*   Pregnant women have an increased incidence of thromboembolism regardless of the mode of delivery.

16   a   *F*   Women with Turner's syndrome have normal external female genitalia.

    b   *F*   In testicular feminisation the phenotype is female but the genotype contains a Y chromosome and testes are present.

    c   *F*   In cryptorchidism the testes have failed to descend and may be in the inguinal canal, but the external genitalia are male.

    d   *T*   The adrenogenital syndrome is the commonest cause of intersex and is caused by a female fetus being exposed to an excess of adrenal androgens.

    e   *F*   Klinefelter's syndrome is a chromosomal disorder with 47XXY composition. The genitalia are male.

17   a   *T*   Because of the increase in plasma volume (approximately 50% in primiparas and 60% in multigravidae) the actual value of electrolytes decreases.

    b   *F*   The mucoid discharge from the cervix *increases* in pregnancy.

    c   *F*   The respiratory tidal volume *increases*, as does the pulmonary blood flow.

    d   *T*   Cardiac output rises in the first trimester and continues to rise until it plateaus at around 34 weeks' gestation.

e *F* In pregnancy a fasting blood glucose less that 5.8 mmol/L is normal and unchanged from the pre-pregnant state.

18 a *F* In severe pre-eclampsia the creatinine clearance rate is reduced.

b *T* The second wave of trophoblastic invasion to form the placental microcirculation is thought to be defective in women with severe PET.

c *T* There is an increased incidence of placental abruption, the placenta itself having reduced perfusion secondary to vasoconstriction.

d *F* The intravascular compartment is *decreased*.

e *T* All levels of electrolytes are increased because the fluid volume in the intravascular compartment is decreased. Rising serum urate levels are used to monitor the disease process.

19 a *F* Once significant antibodies are present there is no point in giving anti-D.

b *T* Amniocentesis can cause Rhesus sensitisation and therefore 250 IU of anti-D are given intramuscularly to Rhesus-negative women (at 20 weeks or less of gestation).

c *F* Anti-D is not given routinely in early pregnancy to Rhesus-negative women.

d *F* The Kleihauer test may not be sensitive enough to pick up a very small transfer of fetal cells into the maternal circulation.

e *F* The ABO incompatibility does not influence initiation of Rhesus disease.

20 a *F* Engagement is defined as when the maximum diameter of the head (the biparietal diameter) has passed through the pelvic brim.

b *F* Engagement is determined by the abdominal findings, as the vaginal level of the presenting part is altered by moulding and therefore is an unreliable finding.

c *T* Engagement is defined as when the maximum diameter of the head (the biparietal diameter) has passed through the pelvic brim.

d *T* In abdominal palpation, engagement is defined as 0/5, 1/5 or 2/5 of the head palpable above the pelvic brim.

e *F* It is the bony parts of the fetal head that are of importance, not the oedema and swelling of the soft tissues of the scalp (caput succedaneum).

21 a *T* In addition to the surge of follicle-stimulating hormone there is a surge in luteinising hormone, the detection of which is used in commercial urine ovulation detector kits.

b *T* As a result of ovulation, the endometrium changes from proliferative to secretory.

c *F* Following ovulation the cervical mucus becomes less fluid and more viscous. It helps prevent the ascent of organisms and sperm to the upper genital tract.

d *T* The basal body temperature rises by approximately 0.3°C following ovulation and remains high throughout the secretory phase.

e *T* The second half of the menstrual cycle is usually constant and is 14 days from ovulation to menstruation. The proliferative phase of the endometrium cycle can vary.

22 a *F* As oestrogen is metabolised through the liver, oral therapy will cause a decrease in antithrombin III. Therefore a woman with a history of thromboembolic disease should be given parenteral therapy, e.g. transdermal or implants.

b *T* Premarin 0.625 mg has been shown to be bone sparing.

c *F* Cystic hyperplasia can be treated medically by giving 12 days of progestogens each month. Repeated endometrial biopsy is warranted.

d *F* An endometrial thickness greater than 5 mm on ultrasound examination is significant in postmenopausal women taking continuous combined oestrogen/progestagen therapy or no therapy.

e *F* Oestrogen replacement therapy will *increase* HDL levels.

23 a *F* If a breech is to be delivered vaginally, then oxytocin should not be used.

b *F* Extraction should never normally be employed. The accoucheur merely guides the delivery of the fetus, which is occurring by uterine contractions and maternal effort.

c *T* This is the widest dimension of the presenting part in a 'frank' or extended breech. It accounts for approximately two-thirds of vaginal breech deliveries.

d *T* In addition to the risks of prematurity, the fetus presenting by the breech has a higher rate of congenital abnormality and ante-partum stillbirth than those with vertex presentation.

e *F* It is important to keep the fetal back anterior otherwise the chin may become caught on the symphysis pubis, causing extension of the head and obstructing delivery.

24 a *F* In the triennial report (2003–5) the maternal mortality rate was 10 per 100 000 total births.

b *F* Deaths related to hypertension are most commonly caused by intracerebral haemorrhage.

c *T* Mendelssohn's syndrome is aspiration of gastric contents and this most commonly occurs after emergency general anaesthesia rather that an elective general or epidural anaesthetic.

d *T* Cardiac disease was the most common cause of indirect death as well as maternal deaths overall. This reflects the growing incidence of acquired heart disease in young women related to poor diets, smoking, alcohol and the growing epidemic of obesity.

e *F* It is very difficult to prevent amniotic fluid embolism.

25 a *T* Hyperprolactinaemia can cause infertility and amenorrhoea. A serum prolactin estimation is an important baseline investigation, even in the woman without galactorrhoea.

b *F* Hyperprolactinaemia is treated with dopamine *agonist* drugs, most commonly bromocriptine or cabergoline.

c *T* Laboratory limits vary and some set the upper limit of normal unrealistically low. The level also increases with stress, eating and nipple stimulation and during sleep, intercourse and anaesthesia.

d *T* Hyperprolactinaemia can be physiological during pregnancy and breast feeding.

e *F* A microadenoma or adenoma of the anterior pituitary gland is often found.

26 a *F* Placebo response rates are in the region of 90%, hence the utmost importance of placebo control in any therapeutic trial.

    b *T* Success has been reported by eating frequent meals, reducing sugar and salt intake and cutting out caffeine sources.

    c *T* A symptom diary together with menstrual dates over the course of two to three months is important to exclude a symptom pattern not in agreement with PMS.

    d *T* The combined oral contraceptive and luteinising hormone releasing hormone (LHRH) agonists have been successfully used in this role.

    e *F* Controlled trials have shown this drug to be successful in improving the symptoms of fatigue, depression, headache, tension and irritability.

27 a *T* Palmar rash is a sign of secondary syphilis, together with the symptoms of fever, headache, bone and joint pains.

    b *F* The primary chancre of syphilis heals after five to eight *weeks*.

    c *F* Condylomata acuminata are warts caused by human papilloma virus; condylomata lata are the classical lesion of *secondary* syphilis.

    d *F* It is with *secondary* disease that the regional lymph nodes become active.

    e *F* Secondary syphilis is highly infective.

28 a *T* Carcinoma of the cervix can be asymptomatic or be associated with intermenstrual, post-coital or postmenopausal bleeding.

    b *T* Stage 1b can be treated with Wertheim's hysterectomy with removal or conservation of the ovaries, depending on the clinical setting and the age of the patient.

    c *F* Adjuvant therapy in carcinoma of the cervix is radiotherapy.

    d *F* The introduction of the cervical screening programme in the UK unfortunately has not decreased the incidence of cervical carcinoma. The rate in younger women (less than 40) is increasing.

e *T* If a fistula develops following local infiltration, then true urinary incontinence can occur.

29 a *F* Polycystic ovarian syndrome is also known as Stein-*Leventhal* syndrome; the clinical symptoms are hirsutism, menstrual problems and obesity.

b *T* If the patient wants to conceive, she may respond to oral clomiphene citrate therapy.

c *F* If the patient's serum testosterone is raised, *hirsutism* may be the presenting complaint.

d *F* Although the plasma LH level is usually increased, the FSH level is low or normal. A follicular phase LH to FSH ratio should be 3 to 1 or more.

e *F* Women with polycystic ovarian syndrome present with *oligomenorrhoea* rather than menorrhagia.

30 a *F* The slowest acceptable rate of progress in a primigravida women is 1 cm every hour and in a multiparous woman 2 cm every hour.

b *F* The commonest cause of delay in labour in a primigravida woman is inefficient uterine action, and oxytocin can be safely used, even in the second stage, once the patient has been assessed.

c *F* In a multiparous woman delay at 7 cm often implies obstructed labour.

d *T* A partogram is a graphic description of labour. Its visual nature conveys much information at a glance.

e *F* Vaginal examinations are normally performed four hourly. It is important that each is documented accurately, together with descent of the head, as palpated per abdomen.

Multiple-choice questions: Paper 4

4

1 Relating to early pregnancy ultrasound scanning.
   a An intrauterine pregnancy sac with a mean sac diameter of 15 mm is in keeping with an anembryonic pregnancy.
   b A positive pregnancy test and no signs of an intrauterine or extrauterine pregnancy or retained products is in keeping with a pregnancy of unknown location.
   c An intrauterine sac with a single fetus measuring 6 mm but no fetal heart pulsation is in keeping with early fetal demise.
   d An incomplete miscarriage is likely when the antero-posterior diameter of the intrauterine echo is 16 mm.
   e Transabdominal scanning with a full bladder is as good as transvaginal scanning.

2 When placenta praevia is suspected at the time of a detailed scan at 20 weeks:
   a a transvaginal scan is more accurate than a transabdominal scan
   b a follow-up scan should be arranged for 26 weeks if the woman remains asymptomatic
   c transvaginal scanning should be avoided in case it provokes vaginal bleeding
   d the risk of subsequent major praevia is 50%
   e 'migration' of the placenta to the upper segment by the third trimester is less likely when the woman has had a previous Caesarean section.

3 Women with suspected placenta praevia should:
   a be managed in hospital if there has been a history of painless ante-partum haemorrhage
   b be delivered by Caesarean section when the placenta is 2 cm from the internal os
   c have a cervical suture inserted to reduce the risk of haemorrhage from dilation of the cervix
   d have a general anaesthetic when planned Caesarean section is undertaken
   e have the Caesarean section operation by a consultant obstetrician if they have had a previous Caesarean section.

4 Relating to cross matching and blood transfusion.
   a Grouping and antibody status should be checked in all pregnant women at booking only.
   b When blood transfusion is considered a possibility, it is not necessary to send a further sample to the laboratory for group and save, if blood group and antibody status are already known.
   c Only Kell negative blood should be used for transfusion in women of childbearing age.
   d In women requiring blood components, only CMV seronegative red cells and platelets should be used.
   e Cross-matched red cells kept in the fridge for women with known major praevia should be replaced every week.

5 Relating to X-linked recessive disorders.
   a There is absence of male to male transmission.
   b The sons of a female carrier have a 50% risk of being affected.
   c The daughters of a female carrier will all be carriers.
   d An affected male will transmit the gene to all his daughters.
   e Heterozygous females may show features of the condition.

6   Fragile X syndrome:
     a   is inherited as an autosomal-dominant condition
     b   is the most common single gene cause of severe mental
         retardation in males
     c   is the most common cause of severe mental retardation
     d   can affect both males and females
     e   means males may carry the affected gene but have normal
         intelligence.

7   Women presenting with:
     a   recurrent genital herpes at the onset of labour will put their
         baby at significant risk of acquiring neonatal herpes if vaginal
         delivery occurs
     b   recurrent genital herpes in the first or second trimesters
         should be delivered by Caesarean section to minimise risk of
         neonatal herpes
     c   a first episode of genital herpes in the first or second trimester
         should be delivered by Caesarean section to minimise risk of
         neonatal herpes
     d   no previous history of genital herpes should be screened for
         type-specific herpes simplex antibodies
     e   primary genital herpes at or just before the onset of labour are
         at greatest risk of perinatal transmission.

8   In cases of suspected pulmonary embolism:
     a   a chest X-ray should be undertaken
     b   the chest X-ray will be abnormal in most cases
     c   when the chest X-ray is normal, bilateral compression duplex
         Doppler ultrasound of the leg veins should be undertaken
     d   if the chest X-ray and leg vein Doppler ultrasound are
         normal, a ventilation-perfusion (V/Q) scan or a computed
         tomography pulmonary angiogram (CTPA) should be
         performed
     e   CTPA has better efficacy compared to a V/Q scan and the
         radiation dose to the fetus is less.

9 Relating to inherited bleeding disorders in pregnancy.
  a Von Willebrand disease is the most common inherited
     bleeding disorder.
  b Von Willebrand disease is inherited as an X-linked recessive
     disorder.
  c Carriers of haemophilia may be at risk of severe bleeding
     complications.
  d Chorion biopsy is the method most widely used in the UK for
     prenatal diagnosis of haemophilia.
  e Clotting-factor levels rise to within normal ranges in carriers
     of haemophilia A.

10 Relating to von Willebrand disease.
  a It has a prevalence of approximately 1%.
  b All three types are due to a defect in von Willebrand factor.
  c Clotting-factor levels rise to within normal ranges in women
     with type 1 von Willebrand disease.
  d Regional anaesthesia is contraindicated.
  e Vaginal delivery is contraindicated.

11 Relating to haemophilia.
  a It is an X-linked recessive disorder.
  b A female fetus will have a 50% chance of being a carrier if the
     mother is a carrier.
  c When parents do not opt for prenatal invasive testing, there is
     no point in trying to sex the pregnancy by ultrasound.
  d The incidence of primary and secondary post-partum
     haemorrhage is not increased in haemophilia carriers.
  e Intranasal desmopressin, a synthetic analogue of vasopressin,
     will increase the plasma concentration of factor VIII.

12 Relating to Rhesus immunoprophylaxis.

 a Anti-D antibodies occur in Rh-negative women when their partner is also Rh-negative.

 b The most important cause of anti-D antibodies is now immunisation during pregnancy where there has been no overt sensitising event.

 c Anti-D immunoglobulin is used in Rhesus-sensitised women to dampen any further antibody response.

 d Anti-D immunoglobulin should always be given within 72 hours of a sensitising event.

 e Anti-D immunoglobulin is not required to be given to Rhesus-negative women who have a spontaneous miscarriage before 12 weeks.

13 Relating to chickenpox.

 a Varicella zoster virus belongs to the herpes group of viruses.

 b The incubation period is seven days.

 c The disease is only infectious once the rash appears.

 d Women from the tropics are more susceptible to chickenpox.

 e Over 90% of UK women are immune to chickenpox.

14 Relating to chickenpox.

 a The varicella zoster virus may reactivate to cause shingles.

 b The varicella vaccine contains live attenuated virus.

 c Pregnant women of unknown immunity who have had contact with chickenpox can be tested, but the result takes at least four days.

 d Pregnant women who have had chickenpox should be given varicella zoster immunoglobulin.

 e Chickenpox is less common in adults and the complications are milder.

15 Women with diabetes:

 a should take folic acid 5 mg daily before conception and up to the 12th week of pregnancy

 b have at least twice the risk of delivering a baby with a major anomaly

c   should ideally have HbA1c levels between 7 and 10% at
    conception
d   are no longer at increased risk of perinatal death following
    the introduction of pre-pregnancy counselling and combined
    obstetric/diabetic clinics
e   have a 40% chance of having a Caesarean section.

16 Recommended methods for cervical priming and induction of
    labour (NICE guideline) include:
a   sweeping the membranes
b   intravenous prostaglandins
c   vaginal prostaglandins in gel form
d   relaxin
e   breast stimulation.

17 The incidence of operative vaginal delivery is reduced:
a   when continuous support is given to women during labour
b   when epidural anaesthesia is used
c   in primiparous women with epidurals when pushing is delayed
    for one to two hours in second stage
d   when a partogram is used
e   if continuous fetal monitoring is used.

18 Relating to continuous fetal heart rate monitoring in labour, the
    pattern is:
a   normal when the baseline rate is 110–160, the variability
    is more than or equal to 5, there are accelerations but no
    decelerations
b   suspicious when the baseline rate is more than 160 but the
    variability is normal and there are no decelerations
c   suspicious when the baseline rate is less than 110 and the
    variability is reduced for 45 minutes
d   pathological when there are late decelerations
e   pathological when the variability has been reduced for more
    than 90 minutes.

19 Regarding ovarian cancer.
  a Multiparous women are at higher risk than nulliparous women.
  b It is the second commonest gynaecological malignancy in most industrialised countries.
  c Peak incidence is about 60 years of age.
  d Secondary tumours in ovary can come from breast, endometrium and cervix.
  e CA125 levels can be raised in ovarian cancer, endometriosis and with peritoneal trauma.

20 Regarding endometrial cancer.
  a Upper-body obesity, carbohydrate intolerance and a personal history of colon cancer are all risk factors.
  b If postmenopausal women have a TVS and there is fluid in the endometrial cavity, malignancy is associated in 25% of cases.
  c FIGO staging for endometrial carcinoma that involves cervical stroma is IIB.
  d Simple hyperplasia coexists with endometrial carcinoma in 25–50% of cases.
  e Endometrial biopsy is the 'gold standard' for making the diagnosis.

21 Regarding recurrent miscarriage.
  a It is worth doing karyotype of both parents, as the incidence of a balanced reciprocal or Robertsonian translocation is around 3–5%.
  b It is defined as consecutive loss of three or more fetuses in the first trimester.
  c It is worth doing a thrombophilia screen because if it is positive, effective treatment is now available.
  d Cervical cerclage is recommended in both recurrent first and second-trimester loss.
  e When no specific abnormalities are found, counselling and reassurance are the mainstays of successful management.

22　Regarding sexually transmitted infections in women.
　　a　Amies and Stuart's transport media are used for culturing gonorrhoea.
　　b　10% of women with gonorrhoea have no symptoms.
　　c　The cervix is the primary site of chlamydial infection.
　　d　Enzyme immunoassay (EIA) is superior at detecting chlamydia compared to a DNA amplification test such as polymerase chain reaction (PCR).
　　e　Chlamydia and gonorrhoea can cause a perihepatitis.

23　Regarding urethral diverticula.
　　a　They commonly present with urinary frequency, urgency and dysuria.
　　b　The imaging of choice is transvaginal scanning.
　　c　They can occur following bladder suspension surgery.
　　d　Antibiotics are the treatment of choice.
　　e　Asymptomatic diverticula should always be treated.

24　Regarding hydatidiform moles.
　　a　In complete moles, all nuclear genes are inherited from the mother.
　　b　The incidence in Asia is highest in the world.
　　c　Most partial moles are haploid.
　　d　In 20% of cases hydatidiform moles develop into choriocarcinoma.
　　e　Pregnancy should be avoided for at least 24 months.

25　Regarding teratogens.
　　a　They can affect the fetus seven days after conception.
　　b　Alcohol consumed by the mother in pregnancy can cause neurodevelopmental abnormalities, including neurosensory hearing loss and poor eye-to-hand coordination.
　　c　Spermicides have been associated with increased chance of birth defects.
　　d　Vitamins are safe in early pregnancy.
　　e　Microwaves should be avoided, as they are non-ionising radiation.

26 Which of the following are contraindicated in a woman who is 35 and a non-smoker with a past history of a deep-vein thrombosis who wants to take the progesterone-only pill for contraception?
   a BMI of 32.
   b Active liver disease.
   c CIN3.
   d History of chlamydia infection.
   e History of endometriosis.

27 The following statements about polycystic ovarian syndrome are true:
   a it is associated with hyperinsulinaemia
   b in resistant cases, it can be treated by ovarian drilling
   c it is associated in later life with hyperplasia of the endometrium
   d it is associated with a low LH
   e when scanning the ovaries there is often a reduced ovarian stroma.

28 Regarding endometriosis.
   a Peak incidence is age 35.
   b It may get worse after the menopause.
   c There is a good correlation between extended disease and severity of symptoms.
   d Surgical treatment is always superior to medical treatment.
   e It can be found in the lung.

29 The following statements are true or false.
   a Patau's syndrome is trisomy 13.
   b Tay-Sachs disease is associated with a single autosomal-recessive gene.
   c Klinefelter's syndrome characteristically is XYY.
   d Cri-du-chat syndrome is due to deletion of part of the long arm of chromosome 5.
   e Achondroplasia is due to an autosomal-recessive gene.

30 The following statements regarding pelvic inflammatory disease are true.

   a If perihepatic adhesions are seen at laparoscopy, the diagnosis is always chlamydia.

   b If the diagnosis of PID is made, an IUCD should be removed.

   c As long as triple therapy is given, follow-up swabs are not needed.

   d Gonorrhoea has now superseded chlamydia as the commonest STI.

   e HSG can cause PID.

Answers: MCQs Paper 4

1 a *F* An anembryonic pregnancy is most likely when the mean sac diameter is more than 20 mm. When it is less than 20 mm the pregnancy is of uncertain viability.

  b *T* This is the correct definition for a pregnancy of unknown location (PUL).

  c *T* This is the correct definition for a silent, delayed or missed miscarriage, also synonymous with early fetal demise.

  d *T* When the maximum antero-posterior diameter is 15 mm or less, genuine retained products are less likely to be confirmed histologically.

  e *F* The imaging quality is not as good, because the pelvic organs will remain further from the transducer.

2 a *T* Transvaginal imaging is more accurate than transabdominal scanning at all gestations in delineating the lower edge in relation to the internal os.

  b *F* A follow-up scan in the second trimester is too soon. A third trimester scan is appropriate. If a major praevia is suspected, a scan at 32 weeks should be performed, and at 36 weeks in cases of minor praevia where the woman remains asymptomatic.

  c *F* Transvaginal scanning has been shown to be safe without risk of bleeding when used with caution and taking into account the possible diagnosis.

  d *F* The risk of subsequent praevia requiring delivery by Caesarean section is only around 10%.

  e *T* 'Migration' is less likely when the placenta is posterior or there has been a previous Caesarean section.

3 a *T* This is recommended best practice (RCOG guideline 27).

  b *T* When the placental edge is within 3 cm of the internal os on ultrasound, the patient should be managed as having a major placenta praevia.

  c *F* There is no evidence to support this practice, which has been tried to reduce bleeding and prolong pregnancy.

  d *F* This is no longer the standard and there is evidence to support the safety of spinal anaesthesia.

   e *T* This is recommended practice because of the high risk of
          major morbidity.

4 a *F* All women should have blood group and antibodies
          checked at booking and 28 weeks.
   b *F* A sample for group and save must be sent to the blood-
          transfusion laboratory if any blood-component therapy is
          contemplated, even if previous blood group and antibody
          status is known.
   c *T* Unless a woman is known to be Kell positive, only Kell
          negative blood should be used because of the risk of
          alloimmunisation.
   d *T* Unless the woman is known to be seropositive,
          seronegative blood components should be used to avoid
          the risk of transmission to the fetus.
   e *T* For women with suspected major placenta praevia, cross-
          matched blood may be kept in the issue fridge. This
          should be replaced every week by newly cross-matched
          units.

5 a *T* An affected father will carry the gene on his X
          chromosome. A son will receive his father's Y sex
          chromosome.
   b *T* A female carrier will transmit the condition to half her
          sons because they will inherit either the affected X or
          unaffected X chromosome.
   c *F* Similarly, the daughters will receive either the affected or
          unaffected X chromosome and so half will be carriers. The
          other healthy X comes from their father.
   d *T* The daughters of an affected male will receive the affected
          X chromosome.
   e *T* This is due to non-random X inactivation resulting in the
          chromosome that carries the affected gene being active in
          most cells.

6 a *F* Fragile X is inherited as an X-linked trait.
   b *T* It is the most common single gene disorder causing
          mental retardation in males.
   c *F* It is the most common single cause of mental retardation
          after Down's syndrome.

d *T* Due to the nature of the fragile X mutation, female carriers may be affected and apparently unaffected males (normal transmitting males) may have the gene.

e *T* Due to the nature of the fragile X mutation, female carriers may be affected and apparently unaffected males (normal transmitting males) may have the gene.

7 a *F* The risk of neonatal herpes is small in women with recurrent genital herpes, because of the presence of protective maternal antibodies.

b *F* A recurrent episode of genital herpes before labour is not an indication for Caesarean section.

c *F* Caesarean section is recommended for all women presenting with first-episode genital lesions at the time of delivery and should be considered in those who present within six weeks of the expected date of delivery.

d *F* In the UK this is not cost-effective due to the low incidence of neonatal herpes (1–2/100 000 live births per annum).

e *T* The risk of neonatal herpes is 40% in women who have primary genital herpes at or just before the onset of labour and the risk is increased when the membranes have been ruptured for more than four hours. If the woman opts for vaginal delivery, invasive procedures such as scalp electrode or fetal blood sampling should be avoided.

8 a *T* A chest X-ray should be performed as the primary investigation and, if normal, compression duplex Doppler of the leg veins should be undertaken.

b *F* The chest X-ray will be normal in more than 50% of proven pulmonary emboli but may detect other pulmonary lesions such as pneumothorax and pneumonia.

c *T* This investigation may diagnose deep venous thrombosis and indirectly confirm pulmonary embolism. Thus further investigation and radiation exposure may not be required.

d *T* Either V/Q scan or CPTA may be undertaken depending on local availability but should be done to make a definitive diagnosis when there is a strong clinical suspicion.

e *T* CTPA has better sensitivity and specificity compared to a V/Q scan, with a lower radiation dose to the fetus but a higher dose to the maternal breasts.

9 a *T* Von Willebrand disease is the most common inherited bleeding disorder, with a prevalence of 1%. Von Willebrand disease, carriers of haemophilia A and B, and factor XI deficiency account for almost 90% of all women with inherited bleeding disorders.

b *F* Types 1 and 2 von Willebrand disease are autosomal dominant and type 3 is autosomal recessive.

c *T* Carriers of haemophilia usually have a clotting-factor level around 50% of normal because they have only one affected chromosome. However, there is a wide range and some have very low factors VIII (haemophilia A) or IX (haemophilia B) and are at risk of severe bleeding complications.

d *T* Chorion biopsy at 11 weeks is the usual method for prenatal diagnosis of haemophilia. Amniocentesis is another option but the diagnosis is later. The uptake rate for invasive testing is not high, because of advances in the management of affected individuals.

e *T* During pregnancy there is a rise in factor VIII in normal women and in carriers of haemophilia A. This is not the case for factor IX and so carriers of haemophilia B may be at risk of bleeding complications.

10 a *T* Von Willebrand disease is the most common inherited bleeding disorder, with a prevalence of 1%. Von Willebrand disease, carriers of haemophilia A and B, and factor XI deficiency account for almost 90% of all women with inherited bleeding disorders.

b *T* All three types are due to a quantitative or qualitative defect in von Willebrand factor. In type 1, there is a partial deficiency of von Willebrand factor. It accounts for 75% and is usually mild. Type 2 is due to a defect in von Willebrand factor. In type 3, there is almost no von Willebrand factor and it is usually severe.

c *T* There is a rise in von Willebrand factor in normal women and in those with type 1 von Willebrand disease.

d *F* If the coagulation screen is normal and factor activity above 50 IU/dl, regional anaesthesia is not contraindicated.

e *F* Scalp electrode, fetal blood sampling, ventouse and difficult forceps deliveries should be avoided. Elective Caesarean section confers no benefit to the neonate.

11 a *T* Both haemophilia A (factor VIII deficiency) and haemophilia B (factor IX deficiency) are X-linked recessive disorders.

b *T* The mother has one abnormal X chromosome and so a female fetus has a 50% chance of being a carrier and a male fetus has a 50% chance of being affected by the condition.

c *F* When a male fetus is identified then the management plan for labour would be altered to avoid fetal scalp electrode, fetal blood sampling, ventouse delivery or difficult forceps delivery.

d *F* There is a rapid fall in factor VIII after delivery, resulting in carriers being at risk of primary and secondary post-partum haemorrhage.

e *T* Desmopressin increases the plasma concentrations of factor VIII and von Willebrand factor by endogenous release.

12 a *F* The development of anti-D antibodies generally results from fetomaternal haemorrhages (FMH) occurring in Rh-negative (dd) women who carry a Rh-positive (Dd or DD) fetus. The father is always Rh-positive, being either homozygous (DD) or heterozygous (Dd).

b *T* Silent fetomaternal haemorrhage may occur in entirely normal pregnancies. However, disruption of the placental bed increases the risk such as in abruption, manual removal of the placenta or stillbirth, but these are usually detected and covered with anti-D.

c *F* Women who are already sensitised should not be given anti-D Ig.

d *T* Anti-D Ig should be given as soon as possible after a sensitising event and always within 72 hours. If it is not given within 72 hours, it may be given up to 10 days but thereafter will not be effective.

e *T* Anti-D Ig should be given to all non-sensitised RhD-negative women who have a surgical evacuation at any gestation or have a spontaneous complete or incomplete abortion after 12 weeks of pregnancy.

13 a *T* Varicella zoster virus is a DNA virus and a member of the herpes family. It is transmitted in respiratory droplets and is very contagious.

b *F* The incubation period is one to three weeks.

c *F* The disease is infectious up to 48 hours before the appearance of the rash and until the vesicles crust over.

d *T* Women from the tropics and subtropics are more likely to be seronegative for varicella zoster virus IgG antibody.

e *T* IgG antibodies to varicella zoster are found in more than 90% of the population, most having acquired immunity in childhood.

14 a *T* Following chickenpox infection, the virus may remain dormant in the sensory nerve root ganglia and reactivate to cause a vesicular skin rash within the distribution of a dermatome. This is known as herpes zoster or shingles.

b *T* The varicella vaccine is live attenuated, and women of reproductive age should avoid pregnancy for three months afterwards.

c *F* Serum can be tested for varicella zoster virus and a result obtained within 24–48 hours. Serum may be available to test from the booking antenatal bloods.

d *F* Varicella zoster immunoglobulin should be given to non-immune pregnant women as soon as possible after significant exposure. This may prevent or attenuate the disease.

e *F* Chickenpox is less common in adults but it is associated with increased morbidity, and maternal death can occur from complications such as pneumonia.

15 a *T* Folic acid reduces the risk of neural tube defects, which are higher in the pregnancies of diabetic women (threefold increase).

b *T* The prevalence of confirmed major anomalies reported to the European Surveillance of Congenital Anomalies was 41.8 per 1000 births in diabetic mothers compared to 21 per 1000 births in general. The increase is primarily due to a higher number of neural tube defects (3.4-fold) and congenital heart disease (3.3-fold).

c *F* The National Service Framework for Diabetes recommends that HbA1c levels should be less than 7% at the time of conception.

d *F* There is a fourfold increase in perinatal mortality in women with diabetes compared to non-diabetic women.

e *F* The Caesarean section rate is almost 60% in diabetic women due to the increased risk of antenatal and intrapartum complications.

16 a *T* Membrane sweeping should be considered whenever induction is offered.

b *F* Intravenous prostaglandins should not be used because of gastrointestinal side effects and hyperstimulation.

c *T* The induction method of choice is prostaglandins, either as gel, tablet or slow-release pessary.

d *F* There is evidence to show that relaxin is ineffective.

e *F* Breast stimulation should not be used because of limited and conflicting evidence.

17 a *T* Continuous support during labour provided by a friend, relative or member of staff reduces the incidence of operative vaginal delivery.

b *F* Epidural analgesia is associated with a higher operative vaginal delivery rate compared to non-epidural methods.

c *T* In primiparous women, delaying pushing for one to two hours in second stage or until there is a strong urge to push reduces the number of mid-cavity and rotational assisted deliveries.

d *T* The use of a partogram leads to fewer operative vaginal deliveries.

e *F* Operative intervention is increased if continuous fetal monitoring is used.

18 a *T* These are the four reassuring features that make the pattern normal.

   b *T* There is one non-reassuring feature and so the pattern is categorised as suspicious.

   c *F* There are two non-reassuring features and the pattern is therefore categorised as pathological.

   d *T* Late decelerations are an abnormal feature and when there is one abnormal feature the pattern is categorised as pathological.

   e *T* Reduced variability for 5–40 minutes is a non-reassuring feature but more than 90 is abnormal and therefore the tracing is pathological.

19 a *F* Nulliparous women are at higher risk as they have more 'ovulation' exposure.

   b *F* Ovarian cancer is the commonest gynaecological malignancy.

   c *F* It occurs predominantly in the fifth to seventh decade of life, with peak age at 75 years.

   d *T* Secondary tumours in the ovary are common and can come from breast and endometrial cancer, and rarely from cervical cancer.

   e *T* CA125 levels are raised in all these conditions but tend to be much higher in ovarian cancer.

20 a *T* All of these are risk factors for endometrial cancer, as are nulliparity and late menopause.

   b *T* Fluid in the endometrial cavity of postmenopausal women should be further investigated with hysteroscopy and biopsy.

   c *T* FIGO staging with endocervical glandular involvement is IIa and cervical stromal involvement is IIB.

   d *F* *Atypical* hyperplasia coexists with endometrial carcinoma in 25–50% of cases.

   e *F* Direct visualisation (hysteroscopy) of the endometrial cavity with biopsy is the 'gold standard'.

21 a *T* The incidence of a balanced reciprocal or Robertsonian translocation is around 3–5%.

b *T* Definition is three or more consecutive miscarriages.

c *F* Recurrent miscarriages have an increased incidence of thrombophilic defects but there is currently no evidence for effective treatment.

d *F* Cervical cerclage is recommended for recurrent second-trimester loss when the diagnosis of cervical incompetence has been made.

e *T* With unexplained recurrent miscarriages, counselling and reassurance are the mainstays of management.

22 a *T* Amies, Stuart's or similar transport media can be used.

b *F* About 50% of women with gonorrhoea and 80% of women with chlamydia will have no symptoms.

c *T* Endocervical swabs rather than HVS must be taken to detect chlamydia.

d *F* Detection rates can be increased to over 90% by PCR compared with EIA for detecting chlamydia.

e *T* Both chlamydia and gonorrhoea can cause Fitz-Hugh-Curtis syndrome.

23 a *T* Urethral diverticula can present with these symptoms as well as the patient being aware of a 'lump'.

b *F* More recently MRI has taken over as the imaging of choice.

c *T* They can occur following surgery but the commonest causes are birth trauma and chronic urethritis.

d *F* Symptomatic urethral diverticula require surgical excision, as currently no successful medical treatment is available.

e *F* Asymptomatic ones do not need treatment.

24 a *F* In most complete moles all nuclear genes are paternal in origin.

b *T* Asia has the highest incidence in the world: 1 in 100 compared to 1 in 1000 in the US.

c *F* Most partial moles are triploid – probably a normal haploid egg fertilised by two sperm.

d *F* In 10–15% of cases, hydatidiform moles may develop into invasive moles.

e *F* Pregnancy should be avoided for 12 months.

25 a   *F*   Teratogens have the ability to affect the fetus about 10–14 days after conception.

     b   *T*   Excess alcohol in pregnancy can cause alcohol syndrome in the fetus.

     c   *F*   Spermicides have not been associated with birth defects.

     d   *F*   Taking extra vitamins (in addition to recommended prenatal vitamins) can be dangerous.

     e   *F*   Microwave ovens are examples of non-ionising radiation, which is not teratogenic.

26 a   *F*   The POP is not contraindicated but the dose should be doubled in women over 70 kg.

     b   *T*   Active liver disease is a contraindication.

     c   *F*   CIN is not a contraindication.

     d   *F*   History of STIs is not a contraindication.

     e   *F*   Progestogens are not contraindicated in endometriosis.

27 a   *T*   In PCOS the underlying metabolic disorder is insulin resistance.

     b   *T*   Ovarian drilling may be effective for PCOS-related subfertility.

     c   *T*   Endometrial hyperplasia and adenocarcinoma are more common in women with PCOS.

     d   *F*   Hormone profile usually shows LH greater than 10 IU/L with raised LH/FSH ratio.

     e   *F*   The ultrasound scan will show increased stromal density, enlarged ovaries and multiple follicular cysts arranged peripherally around the ovary.

28 a   *F*   Peak incidence is in the early 40s.

     b   *F*   With lack of oestrogen stimulation of endometriosis decreases.

     c   *F*   There is a poor correlation of extent of disease to severity of symptoms.

     d   *F*   Surgical treatment and medical treatment have not been directly compared effectively.

     e   *T*   Endometriosis can occur at sites outside the pelvis.

29 a *T* Patau's syndrome is trisomy 13. Down's syndrome is trisomy 21, Edward's syndrome is trisomy 18.

   b *T* Tay-Sachs disease is a single autosomal-recessive gene.

   c *F* Klinefelter's is XXY.

   d *F* Cri-du-chat is deletion of part of the short arm of chromosome 5.

   e *F* Achondroplasia is due to an autosomal-dominant gene.

30 a *F* Fitz-Hugh-Curtis syndrome can also be caused by gonorrhoea.

   b *F* The IUCD may be left in place and appropriate antibiotics may be given.

   c *F* Follow-up swabs are always needed after therapy.

   d *F* Currently the commonest STI in women is chlamydia.

   e *T* Hysterosalpingogram can introduce infection and cause pelvic inflammatory disease.

Single best answers: obstetrics

1 One of the following statements is false.
Chickenpox in pregnancy:
  a may become complicated and result in maternal death
  b can be acquired from contact with shingles
  c tends to be more complicated at later gestations
  d should be treated with oral acyclovir within 24 hours of the onset of the rash
  e can be alleviated with varicella zoster immunoglobulin.

2 One of the following statements is true.
Genital herpes in pregnancy:
  a can be acquired from contact with shingles
  b if recurrent has a strong association with neonatal herpes
  c if acquired for the first time at 35 weeks, vaginal delivery should be considered
  d may be caused by herpes simplex type 1 (HSV-1) or herpes simplex type 2 (HSV-2)
  e is low risk to the baby if it has been acquired for the first time at the onset of labour.

3   One of the following statements is false.
    Relating to thromboembolism.
    a   Venous thromboembolism (VTE) is 10 times more common
        in the pregnant woman compared to the non-pregnant
        woman of comparable age.
    b   The risk of VTE is four times higher in the puerperium
        compared to the antenatal period.
    c   A positive D-dimer test in pregnancy is consistent with VTE.
    d   When pulmonary thromboembolism is suspected, both a V/Q
        scan and bilateral Doppler ultrasound leg studies should be
        performed.
    e   The incidence of post-thrombotic syndrome is reduced by
        wearing graduated elastic compression stockings for two years
        after the acute event.

4   One of the following is false.
    Relating to obstetric anal sphincter injury.
    a   Anal sphincter injury complicates 1% of all vaginal deliveries.
    b   Sonographic abnormalities of the anal sphincter anatomy have
        been identified in one-third of women after vaginal delivery.
    c   A third-degree tear involves partial or complete disruption
        of the external and internal anal sphincters but not the anal
        epithelium.
    d   A fourth-degree tear involves injury to the anal sphincter
        complex and the anal epithelium.
    e   Obstetric anal sphincter injury includes both second and
        third-degree tears.

5   One of the following is true.
    Relating to post-operative management of obstetric anal
    sphincter injury.
    a   Broad-spectrum antibiotics should be used.
    b   Loperamide should be used to reduce frequency of bowel
        motion.
    c   Pelvic floor exercises are contraindicated.

d 60–80% of women will have incontinence of flatus and faecal urgency at 12 months.

e Residual defects seen on endoanal ultrasound should be repaired.

6 One of the following statements is false.
In diabetic pregnancy:

a insulin requirements increase in the second and third trimesters

b glucose levels should be maintained between 5.5 (fasting) and 7.0 mmol/L (post-prandial)

c glycosylated haemoglobin should be less than 7%

d insulin requirement will remain the same until two weeks after delivery

e ketoacidosis is associated with a high fetal mortality.

7 One of the following statements is false.
In severe pre-eclampsia, the following may occur:

a abnormal liver enzymes

b cholestasis

c epigastric pain

d liver tenderness

e HELLP syndrome.

8 One of the following statements is false.
In the management of severe pre-eclampsia:

a antihypertensive treatment should be commenced when the diastolic blood pressure is over 110 mm Hg

b antihypertensive treatment should be commenced when the systolic blood pressure is over 160 mm Hg

c angiotensin-converting enzyme (ACE) inhibitors are ideal for control of moderate hypertension

d labetalol, given orally or intravenously, is useful for the acute management of severe hypertension

e nifedipine, given orally, is useful for the acute management of severe hypertension.

9 One of the following is true.

In the management of severe pre-eclampsia in the postnatal period:

a antihypertensive treatment should be stopped immediately after delivery

b severe pre-eclampsia does not present in the postnatal period

c eclampsia can occur up to four weeks postnatally

d persisting hypertension and proteinuria at six weeks does not require investigation for underlying renal disease

e atenolol is contraindicated in women planning to breast feed.

10 One of the following is false.

A woman with a breech presentation at term should be advised that:

a planned Caesarean section carries a reduced perinatal mortality and early neonatal morbidity compared to planned vaginal birth

b planned Caesarean section carries a slightly increased risk of immediate complications compared to planned vaginal birth

c planned Caesarean section carries no additional risk to her health in the long term, outside pregnancy

d the long-term health of her baby will be influenced by mode of delivery

e routine X-ray pelvimetry will not be undertaken if vaginal delivery is anticipated.

11 One of the following is true.

Relating to cord presentation and prolapse.

a Cord presentation may be reliably predicted by routine ultrasound scanning in the third trimester.

b In the presence of a normal fetal heart rate pattern, cord prolapse is not possible.

c When cord prolapse occurs in labour, Caesarean section is required.

d Cord prolapse should be suspected when variable decelerations occur soon after membrane rupture.

e Cord prolapse is unlikely when the lie is unstable.

12 One of the following is true.
   In women with breech presentation at term:

   a the perinatal mortality is lower when vaginal delivery is planned compared to when Caesarean section is planned

   b the neonatal morbidity in the first week of life is higher when vaginal delivery is planned compared to when Caesarean section is planned

   c the long-term health of the babies delivered vaginally is worse than those delivered by Caesarean section

   d planned Caesarean section compared to planned vaginal birth is associated with additional risks to long-term maternal health

   e planned Caesarean section compared to planned vaginal birth is associated with no additional risk of immediate serious complications.

13 One of the following is false.
   Clinical features of pre-eclampsia include:

   a severe headache

   b nystagmus

   c epigastric pain

   d liver tenderness

   e abnormal liver enzymes.

14 One of the following is false.
   A primiparous woman at 32 weeks has a persistently elevated blood pressure of 165/115. Which of the following would you not give?

   a oral labetalol

   b intravenous labetalol

   c oral nifedipine

   d sublingual nifedipine

   e intravenous hydralazine.

15 One of the following is false.

In a woman with severe pre-eclampsia:

a magnesium sulphate should be used when there is a significant risk of eclampsia

b magnesium sulphate is the treatment of choice to control seizures

c antihypertensive treatment should be commenced when the systolic blood pressure is more than 160 mm

d fluids should be restricted to 80 mL/hour

e syntometrine should be given for prevention of haemorrhage for management of the third stage.

16 One of the following is false.

The following are associated with cord prolapse:

a preterm labour

b fetal abnormality

c occipito-transverse position

d internal podalic version

e artificial rupture of the membranes.

17 One of the following is false.

In a woman with placenta praevia:

a a morbidly adherent placenta is more likely when the placenta is anterior and there has been a previous Caesarean section

b a spinal anaesthetic is contraindicated for delivery by Caesarean section

c there is no evidence to support the use of autologous transfusion

d cell salvage has a place in management

e cervical cerclage is not recommended.

18 One of the following is false.

The following are contraindicated when vaginal breech birth is being considered:

a previous Caesarean section

b footling breech

c breech presentation first diagnosed in labour

d estimated fetal size more than 4 kg

e a growth-restricted fetus at term estimated at less than 2 kg.

19 One of the following is false.

Relating to the pre-pregnancy management of women with diabetes.

 a The longer the woman has had diabetes, the greater the risk of pregnancy complications.

 b Folic acid 5 mg should be taken pre-pregnancy until 12 weeks' gestation.

 c The HbA1c level should be maintained below 6.1%.

 d Oral hypoglycaemic medication should be discontinued pre-pregnancy and substituted with insulin.

 e Rapid-acting insulin analogues (aspart and lispro) may adversely affect the fetus.

20 One of the following is false.

Relating to gestational diabetes.

 a A body mass index of more than 30 kg/m^2 at booking is a risk factor for gestational diabetes.

 b Screening for gestational diabetes is undertaken using glucose urinalysis.

 c Women who have had previous gestational diabetes should be offered a glucose tolerance test after the first trimester.

 d In women with gestational diabetes, good glycaemic control will reduce the risk of macrosomia.

 e If diet and exercise fail to control adequate blood glucose levels, an oral hypoglycaemic agent may be necessary.

21 One of the following is true.

Relating to the management of diabetes during pregnancy.

 a Rapid-acting insulin analogues (aspart and lispro) have no advantages over soluble human insulin during pregnancy.

 b After the first trimester, women should be advised that there is risk of hypoglycaemia.

 c Diabetic retinopathy is a contraindication to vaginal birth.

 d Routine monitoring of fetal well-being is not recommended before 38 weeks unless there is suspected intrauterine growth restriction.

 e Diabetic retinopathy is a contraindication to rapid optimisation of blood glucose levels in the presence of a high HbA1c.

22 One of the following is false.

Relating to group B streptococcus (GBS).

a   GBS is the most frequent cause of severe early-onset infection in neonates.

b   Routine screening for antenatal GBS is recommended.

c   There is insufficient evidence for intrapartum antibiotic administration in women who have been found to have carried GBS in a previous pregnancy.

d   Intrapartum antibiotics are recommended to women who have had a previous neonate with GBS.

e   In women with preterm rupture of the membranes, GBS antibiotic prophylaxis is not necessary.

23 One of the following is false.

Relating to intrapartum fetal heart rate monitoring.

a   The normal range for the baseline fetal heart rate is 110–160.

b   The baseline variability is normally more than five beats per minute.

c   When the baseline variability has been reduced for 90 minutes or more, the tracing is categorised as pathological.

d   The presence of late decelerations is in keeping with hypoxia.

e   Even when variable decelerations occur as the only non-reassuring feature, a fetal blood sample should be undertaken.

24 One of the following is true.

When categorising fetal rate pattern features into reassuring, non-reassuring and abnormal:

a   a baseline rate of 105 is reassuring

b   a single prolonged deceleration lasting up to three minutes is abnormal

c   early decelerations are abnormal

d   variable decelerations are non-reassuring

e   baseline variability of less than five for 30 minutes is non-reassuring.

25 One of the following is false.

In the assessment of intrauterine growth restriction:

a   the measurement of the abdominal circumference is the single most reliable ultrasonic parameter b an amniotic single pool depth of less than 2 cm is abnormal

   c a cardiotocograph showing no accelerations over a period of 40 minutes is abnormal

   d absent end diastolic flow in the Doppler assessment of the umbilical artery is abnormal

   e the diagnosis is suspected when the fetal head circumference measurement is less than the 10th centile.

26 One of the following is false.
Relating to smoking and substance misuse.

   a Smoking in pregnancy is associated with low birthweight.

   b Smoking in pregnancy is associated with an increased risk of sudden infant death syndrome.

   c Smoking in pregnancy is associated with an increased risk of pre-eclampsia.

   d Cocaine use in pregnancy is associated with abruption.

   e Alcohol is a teratogen.

27 One of the following is true.
Relating to shoulder dystocia.

   a The recurrence risk is 50%.

   b Half of all shoulder dystocia cases occur when the babies have a normal birthweight.

   c Macrosomia can be reliably predicted antenatally.

   d Early induction in cases of suspected macrosomia has been shown to reduce the risk of shoulder dystocia.

   e The size of the pelvic outlet in association with the perineum contributes to the mechanism of shoulder dystocia.

28 One of the following is false.
In women with obstetric cholestasis:

   a the risk of stillbirth is unclear if no intervention is undertaken

   b the current stillbirth rate for obstetric cholestasis is the same as the general population risk

   c the incidence of preterm delivery is higher

   d intrauterine growth restriction is more common

   e the risk of fetal death does not correlate with the derangement in liver function tests.

29 One of the following is true.

The requirement for operative vaginal delivery:

a is reduced with the use of epidural analgesia

b is increased when pushing is delayed in second stage in primiparous women with epidural analgesia

c is increased when women labour in the upright or lateral positions

d is increased when a partogram is used

e is decreased with the use of oxytocin in primiparous women with epidurals.

30 One of the following is false.

Relating to types of operative delivery.

a An outlet forceps is defined as such when the fetal head is at or on the perineum at application.

b A low-cavity forceps delivery is defined as such when the leading point of the fetal head is 2 cm or more below the ischial spines at application.

c A mid-cavity forceps is defined as such when the leading point of the fetal head is at the level of the ischial spines or up to 2 cm below at application.

d A mid-cavity forceps is when the head is one-fifth palpable abdominally.

e A high-cavity forceps is used for delivery of a second twin.

Answers: Single best answers: obstetrics

1 e

Varicella immunoglobulin has no therapeutic benefit once chickenpox has developed.

2 d

Shingles is caused by varicella virus, not herpes. The risks to the neonate are small in women presenting with recurrent herpes at the onset of labour. When first-episode genital herpes is acquired within six weeks of delivery, then Caesarean section should be considered. Primary rather than recurrent genital herpes is a significant risk factor for neonatal herpes.

3 c

D-dimer testing should not be used in pregnant women, because of the high rate of false positive results. This is due to physiological changes in the coagulation system resulting in elevated D-dimer levels in pregnancy.

4 e

A second-degree tear involves the perineal muscles but does not involve the anal sphincter.

5 a

Laxatives are recommended, not antidiarrhoeal agents. Physiotherapy and pelvic floor exercises are advised for 6–12 weeks after repair. Sixty to 80% will be asymptomatic at 12 months. Residual defects do not require repair if the woman is asymptomatic.

6 d

Insulin requirements fall immediately after delivery.

7 b

Cholestasis in not a feature of pre-eclampsia.

8 c

ACE inhibitors, angiotensin receptor-blocking (ARB) drugs diuretics and atenolol should be avoided in the control of blood pressure in women with severe pre-eclampsia.

9 c

Anti-hypertensive treatment must be continued in the postnatal period. Pre-eclampsia can present for the first time in the postnatal period and eclampsia can occur up to four weeks after delivery. Forty per cent of cases of eclampsia occur post-partum. The blood pressure may take up to three months to return to normal after pre-eclampsia but persistent proteinuria and hypertension may reflect underlying renal disease.

10 d

The long-term health of the baby is not influenced by the mode of delivery. All the rest are true.

11 d

Routine ultrasound in the third trimester cannot reliably predict cord presentation. Cord prolapse can be present when the fetal heart rate pattern is normal but is typically associated with variable decelerations. If cord prolapse is diagnosed at full dilatation, vaginal delivery is possible. An unstable lie is a risk factor for cord prolapse.

12 b

In women with breech presentation at term, the perinatal mortality and early neonatal morbidity is higher when vaginal delivery is planned compared to when Caesarean section is planned. There is no evidence that the long-term health of babies delivered at term is influenced by the mode of delivery. There are no long-term maternal health issues relating to planned Caesarean section compared to planned vaginal birth, but there is the additional risk of immediate complications when Caesarean section is undertaken.

13 b

Nystagmus is not a presenting feature of pre-eclampsia.

14 d

Sublingual nifedipine can cause a rapid fall in blood pressure and is contraindicated.

15 e

Syntometrine contains syntocinon and ergometrine. Ergometrine raises blood pressure and is contraindicated.

16 c

There is no association between cord prolapse and occipito-transverse position.

17 b

There is increasing experience in the use of spinal anaesthesia for delivery by Caesarean section in women with placenta praevia.

18 c

There is no absolute contraindication to anticipate vaginal breech delivery when a breech presentation is first diagnosed in labour.

19 e

Rapidly acting insulin analogues have advantages over soluble human insulin and have no adverse effect on the fetus.

20 b

Glucose urinalysis is an ineffective method of screening for gestational diabetes.

21 d

Rapid-acting insulin analogues are as effective as soluble human insulin, with no disadvantages. Diabetic women should be advised of the risk of hypoglycaemia, particularly during the first trimester. Vaginal delivery is not contraindicated in the presence of diabetic retinopathy. Diabetic retinopathy should not be considered a contraindication to rapid blood glucose level control.

22 b

Routine screening (either bacteriological or risk-based) for antenatal GBS is not recommended.

23 e

Usually two or more non-reassuring features or one or more abnormal features are required before a tracing is categorised as pathological. Action is then required either with a fetal blood sample to assess pH or with immediate delivery. If there is only one non-reassuring feature, such as variable decelerations, it is appropriate simply to continue to observe the tracing (NICE guideline 55, Intrapartum Care 2007).

24 d

A baseline rate of 110–160 is reassuring. A single prolonged deceleration up to three minutes is non-reassuring; more than three minutes is abnormal. Early decelerations are non-reassuring. Baseline variability of less than five for more than 40 minutes but less than 90 minutes is non-reassuring; 90 minutes or more is abnormal.

25 e

Measurement of the head circumference alone is inadequate to make the diagnosis of intrauterine growth restriction.

26 c

For unknown reasons pre-eclampsia is less common in smokers. The incidence of alcohol-related birth defects and the fetal alcohol syndrome increases sharply in women who consume more than three units per day.

27 b

The recurrence risk is 10%. The range of error for ultrasonic estimate of fetal weight is 10% and up to 20% for macrosomic fetuses. There is no evidence at present to support early induction. The pelvic outlet is not a significant factor, and an episiotomy is performed or extended to allow better access for vaginal manipulations.

28 d

Recent data does not show an increase in the stillbirth rate compared to the general population. Preterm delivery, both iatrogenic and spontaneous, is higher but intrauterine growth restriction is not associated with cholestasis. There is no proven link between risk of fetal death and level of derangement of liver function tests.

29 e

Epidural analgesia increases the need for operative vaginal delivery. Delayed pushing reduces the need for forceps delivery in primiparous women with epidurals. Upright or lateral positions and the use of a partogram all decrease the need for operative vaginal delivery.

30 e

There is no place for high forceps deliveries in modern obstetric practice.

Single best answers: gynaecology

6

1   A 48-year-old woman presents with intermenstrual bleeding for
    two months and episodes of bleeding occurring any time in the
    cycle. There is no associated pain.
    Differential diagnosis for intermenstrual bleeding does not
    include:
    a   endocervical polyp
    b   cervical malignancy
    c   endometrial polyp
    d   ovarian teratoma
    e   atrophic vaginitis.

2   All of the following drugs are associated with
    hyperprolactinaemia, apart from:
    a   reserpine
    b   progesterone-only contraceptive pill
    c   methyldopa
    d   ranitidine
    e   chlorpromazine.

3   All of the following are effects of premature menopause, apart
    from:
    a   decreased cardiovascular risk
    b   infertility
    c   osteoporosis
    d   vasomotor symptoms
    e   vaginal dryness.

4   A 32-year-old woman presents to the gynaecology clinic with infrequent periods. A hormone profile is done and all of the following are consistent with polycystic ovarian syndrome, apart from:

a   increased androgen levels
b   normal FSH
c   normal oestradiol
d   decreased LH
e   low progesterone levels.

5   A 28-year-old woman attends the colposcopy clinic after an abnormal smear test. The smear is reported as severe dyskaryosis and she has an intrauterine contraceptive device *in situ*. All of the following statements are likely to be true, apart from:

a   the cervix is macroscopically normal
b   acetic acid is applied and an irregular white area is apparent to the left of the cervical os
c   Lugol's iodine is applied and the same area stains dark brown while the rest of the cervix stains pale
d   a biopsy is taken
e   the IUCD can stay, as it will not aggravate the cervical abnormality.

6   A 24-year-old woman presents with the absence of periods for nine months. She started her periods at the age of 13 years and had a regular 28-day cycle until 18 months ago. The periods then became irregular, occurring every two to three months until they stopped completely. The following are all included in the differential diagnosis of secondary amenorrhoea, apart from:

a   excessive exercise
b   hyperprolactinaemia
c   hyperthyroidism
d   premature ovarian failure
e   significant weight loss

7 The following statements regarding adenomyosis are true, apart from one.
   a It tends to occur in women over 35 years.
   b Risk factors include increased parity, termination and quick labours.
   c The condition commonly occurs in association with endometriosis.
   d With each period, bleeding occurs from the endometrial tissue into the smooth muscle.
   e The diagnosis can be made by ultrasound or magnetic resonance imaging scan.

8 A 20-year-old woman is referred with a problem of post-coital bleeding. Over the past two months it has occurred on six occasions and there has been a small amount of bright red blood noticed after intercourse. There is no associated pain. The following investigations should initially be performed, apart from:
   a cervical smear
   b endocervical swab for chlamydia
   c colposcopy
   d endocervical swab for gonorrhoea
   e speculum examination to observe the cervix.

9 The following are all consistent with the diagnosis of antiphospholipid syndrome except:
   a hydatidiform mole
   b severe early-onset pre-eclampsia
   c arterial or venous thrombosis
   d mid-trimester fetal loss
   e placental abruption.

10 The following are all causes of recurrent miscarriage, apart from:
   a parental chromosomal abnormality
   b activated protein C-resistance
   c uncontrolled hypothyroidism

    d chlamydia infection

    e submucosal fibroids.

11 Which one of the following statements about pituitary tumours is true?

    a Weight loss is a common feature of pituitary failure (hypopituitarism) due to a pituitary tumour.

    b Visual field loss in female patients with prolactin-secreting pituitary tumours (prolactinoma) is usual.

    c Adrenocorticotrophic hormone (ACTH) secreting pituitary tumours cause a syndrome of cortisol excess that can lead to exaggerated vertical growth in adolescence.

    d Growth hormone deficiency is a recognised feature in adult patients presenting with acromegaly due to a pituitary macroadenoma.

    e A low testosterone level is more common than a low thyroxine level in men with non-functioning gonads.

12 Which of the following statements concerning the anterior pituitary is true?

    a It develops in the embryo from a down-growth of the hypothalamus.

    b It secretes antidiuretic hormone (ADH).

    c It is regulated by hypothalamic-releasing hormones.

    d It secretes its hormones into the pituitary portal system.

    e It is down-regulated by low oestrogen levels.

13 Which one of the following statements about the implantation of the human embryo is true?

    a It will occur at any time over a period of about 14 days.

    b It will occur whether or not the zona pellucida is present.

    c It will occur when the cytotrophoblast contacts the endometrial epithelium and begins to invade the maternal tissue.

    d It will occur with the inner cell mass closest to the endometrium.

    e It will occur even if there is only cytotrophoblast present.

14 Which one of the following statements about puberty is true?
   a Puberty is preceded by falling plasma levels of adrenal androgens.
   b The first menstrual period is called the adrenarche.
   c The pubertal growth spurt is the first sign of puberty.
   d Pubic hair growth is stimulated in girls by oestrogen.
   e Spermatogenesis starts at puberty.

15 Which is the most appropriate statement concerning pulmonary embolism?
   a It is now rarely fatal, with the introduction of modern diagnostic tests and treatments.
   b It gives an area of lung which is unventilated on a ventilation-perfusion scan.
   c It does not usually show up on a CT pulmonary angiogram.
   d It is likely that the patient has symptoms of deep-vein thrombosis.
   e It may give symptoms similar to pneumonia.

16 One of the following is true. It is recognised that the positive predictive value of initial mammography for breast cancer within the national screening programme in the UK is 16%. This means that:
   a 16% of people who have breast cancer are detected on initial mammography
   b 84% of people without breast cancer have a normal mammogram
   c 16% of initial mammograms are abnormal
   d a patient with an abnormal initial mammogram has a 16% chance of having breast cancer
   e out of every 100 patients with an abnormal mammogram, 16 will develop breast cancer by the time they have their next screening programme.

17 One of the following is true. Successful fertilisation and subsequent normal embryonic development:
   a require at least two spermatozoa
   b require the retention of the cortical granules in the oocyte

    c are most likely when the oocytes have been ovulated in an immature stage

    d require exclusion of the second polar body

    e often occur when the oocyte has lost its zona pellucida.

18 One of the following is true. The increase in maternal blood volume in pregnancy occurs as a result of:

    a peripheral vasoconstriction

    b a reduction in progesterone

    c decreased synthesis of vasopressin

    d increased aldosterone synthesis

    e reduced renin activity.

19 One of the following is true. Decreased peripheral resistance in pregnancy has been attributed to an increase in synthesis of:

    a angiotensin

    b endothelin

    c nitric oxide

    d renin

    e thromboxane.

20 A 25-year-old woman on liver enzyme inducers is requesting contraceptive advice. The method providing her with the most reliable form of contraception would be:

    a combined oral contraceptive pill

    b Depo-Provera injection

    c diaphragm

    d male condom

    e progesterone-only pill.

21 A 35-year-old woman comes requesting long-term reversible contraception. You advise that the method that can provide the longest protection is:

    a contraceptive implant

    b copper intrauterine device

    c Depo-Provera injection

    d intrauterine hormonal system (IUS)

    e laparoscopic sterilisation.

22 Regarding cervical cancer, which is the true statement?
  a HPV types 6 and 12 are high risk for developing cervical cancer.
  b The new vaccines can prevent invasive carcinoma but not CIN.
  c As soon as the new vaccination is introduced, cervical screening programmes can cease.
  d HPV types 16 and 18 account for the majority of cervical cancer in the UK.
  e HPV is an oncogenic virus for squamous cell but not adenocarcinoma of the cervix.

23 Regarding the menstrual cycle, which is the true statement?
  a Menstruation occurs with vasodilation of the spiral arteries.
  b The LH surge triggers menstruation.
  c The Graafian follicle develops during the luteal phase.
  d Both the follicle and the corpus luteum secrete oestradiol.
  e Progesterone levels fall after the onset of menstruation.

24 Regarding Müllerian duct abnormalities which is the true statement?
  a occur about 1 in 500
  b the commonest uterine abnormality is septate uterus
  c occur not infrequently with gastrointestinal abnormalities
  d surgical correction of a septate uterus is followed by fetal salvage in <60% of cases
  e longitudinal vaginal septa are more common than transverse ones.

25 Choose the correct statement: Uterine leiomyosarcomas:
  a are associated with exposure to tamoxifen
  b originate from leiomyomas
  c pelvic radiotherapy has a significant impact on survival
  d commonly metastasise to the brain
  e anthracycline-based chemotherapy has no place in treatment.

26 Which one of the following statements about the menopause is correct?
   a Progesterone levels rise after the menopause.
   b LH levels rise after the menopause.
   c The pituitary stops secreting LH and FSH at the menopause.
   d Menstrual cycles remain regular until the last menstrual period.
   e The number of oocytes in the ovary remains constant until the menopause.

27 Choose the correct statement: The female reproductive tract plays important roles in sperm transport by:
   a trapping most spermatozoa in the cervical crypt for many days
   b regulating sperm transport so that cells reach the site of fertilisation around the time of ovulation
   c allowing sperm transport at all stages of the ovarian cycle
   d preventing spermatozoa from swimming out of the peritoneal cavity
   e providing an acidic environment to keep the spermatozoa active.

28 Which one of the following statements is true: Semen analysis:
   a identifies men with high-quality fertile spermatozoa
   b identifies men with low sperm concentrations that might affect fertility
   c can always be used to predict fertility
   d cannot identify abnormal spermatozoa
   e identifies men with hypopituitarism.

29 One of the following is true. A malignant tumour arising in the mesenchymal tissue is called:
   a adenoma
   b carcinoma
   c lymphoma
   d melanoma
   e sarcoma.

30 One of the following is true. Affording moral status to a human embryo/fetus means that it now has:

a an inalienable right to life
b a right to life
c a right to consideration
d a right dependent on moral consensus
e a right not to be harmed.

Answers: Single best answers: gynaecology

1 d

Teratomas are also known as dermoid cysts. They occur in the ovary and are not related to intermenstrual bleeding.

2 b

The progesterone-only and combined oral contraceptive pills are not associated with hyperprolactinaemia.

3 a

Premature menopause (before the age of 40 years) occurs in 1% of women and has significant physical and psychological consequences. When ovarian failure occurs, there is an increased cardiovascular risk.

4 d

With polycystic ovarian syndrome, anovulation occurs and there are increased androgen levels and increased LH:FSH ratio. Therefore, decreased LH is not consistent with polycystic ovary disease.

5 c

Abnormal tissue stains white with acetic acid because abnormal cells have high density nuclei which take up the acetic acid more than normal cells. In contrast, abnormal cells have lower glycogen content than normal cells and stain less well, remaining pale when iodine is applied.

6 c

When considering the causes of secondary amenorrhoea, one should think of causes in the following categories: hypothalamic, pituitary, ovarian or uterine. When considering the pituitary causes, hyperprolactinaemia (e.g. drugs, tumour), breast feeding or hypothyroidism – not hyperthyroidism – are causes.

7 b

Risk factors include increased parity, termination and previous Caesarean section; history of quick labours is not a risk factor. This is a benign condition whereby functioning endometrial glands and stroma are found within the endometrium. Classically the diagnosis may only be made histologically after hysterectomy for dysmenorrhoea. The prevalence of adenomyosis is unknown, as diagnosis is only confirmed by hysterectomy. It is a cause of menorrhagia and dysmenorrhoea.

8 c

A sexually transmitted infection screen should be performed and a cervical smear should also be taken to detect any dyskaryosis, but colposcopy would not be a first-line investigation and would only be performed if the cervical smear was abnormal.

9 a

Hydatidiform mole is not associated with antiphospholipid syndrome.

10 d

Chlamydia infection is not associated with recurrent miscarriage, but bacterial vaginosis can be associated with second-trimester loss. Only a minority of women with recurrent miscarriage will have a cause identified.

11 e

Pituitary failure in women can be caused by tumours, trauma or infarction. It can present with amenorrhoea, loss of libido, reduced pubic and axillary hair, mild adrenal deficiency, secondary myxoedema and hypoglycaemic episodes. Growth hormone excess is usually related to an eosinophil adenoma of the pituitary.

12 c

The anterior pituitary arises from an invagination of the oral ectoderm. It secretes ACTH, FSH, GH, LH, PRL and TSH. It is regulated by hormones from the hypothalamus.

13 d

Implantation occurs approximately seven days after fertilisation and is initiated when the blastocyst comes into contact with the uterine wall.

14 a

Thelarche is the first sexual change to occur, with development of the breast. Then adrenarche – pubic and then axillary hair growth, which are dependent on adrenal development. The final

manifestation of sexual maturity is the onset of menstruation
– menarche.

15 e

Pulmonary embolism remains a common cause of death, and a
V/Q scan may show an underperfused area. CTPA is superior
to V/Q scans in detecting emboli. Symptoms are sudden onset
dyspnea, tachypnoea, chest pain, cough and haemoptysis.

16 d

17 d

Sperm stimulate a change in the zona pellucida that prevents
further sperm entering the cell and stimulate the second meiotic
division in the egg with subsequent production of the second
polar body.

18 d

In pregnancy there is an increase in cardiac output and a decrease
in peripheral vascular resistance. Progesterone concentrations
rise.

19 c

20 b

Depo-Provera is not metabolised through the liver and has a
failure rate of 0.1–1.2 per 100 women years.

21 b

Copper IUCDs can be left for five to 12 years and intrauterine
hormonal systems for five years.

22 d

HPV types 16 and 18 cause 70% of cervical cancers. There is
now a vaccine for HPV which is intended for females from the
age of 10 upwards.

23 d

At the end of the luteal phase, the corpus luteum regresses,
causing a decrease in oestrogen and progesterone production.
This is followed by intense spasmodic contraction of the spiral
section of the endometrial arterioles, giving rise to ischaemic
necrosis, and the endometrium is shed.

24 b

Müllerian duct abnormalities occur with the frequency of about 1 in 5000. They commonly occur in association with renal tract abnormalities and surgical correction of a septate uterus is followed by fetal salvage in nearly 90% of cases.

25 a

Uterine fibroids are not generally thought to develop into leiomyosarcomas. Adjuvant pelvic radiotherapy may reduce local recurrence rate, but there has not been proven significant impact on overall survival. They commonly metastasise to the lungs. Anthracycline-based chemotherapy has a role in treatment.

26 b

Menopause is defined as the last menstrual period and, prior to this, hormonal changes will occur. The ovarian production of oestradiol decreases, causing FSH and LH, which are produced from the pituitary, to rise. Prior to the last menstrual period the menstrual cycles may be irregular. The number of oocytes decreases throughout a lifetime and even starts decreasing in the female fetus.

27 b

Once deposited in the vagina, sperm move quickly to avoid the acidic environment and are filtered by the cervical mucus. A small proportion move into the uterine cavity, where their progress is aided by uterine muscular contractions. Some then proceed through the uterotubal junction and then reside in a reservoir in the fallopian tube. At ovulation the sperm become capacitated and hyperactivated and proceed to the tubal ampulla.

28 b

Semen analysis provides information about the amount of semen that a man produces and the number and quality of sperm.

29 e

An adenoma is of glandular origin and a melanoma is a malignant tumour of melanocytes.

30 d

Ethical issues are always up for debate in O and G and cannot be avoided!

7

Extended matching questions: obstetrics

1 *Options*

    a Commence low molecular weight heparin (LMWH).

    b Commence warfarin.

    c Continue warfarin.

    d Change warfarin to LMWH.

    e Commence LMWH after delivery.

    f Give support stockings only.

    g Continue LMWH.

    h Change from LMWH to warfarin.

Instructions

You are required to choose the single most appropriate form of thromboprophylaxis for each pregnancy-associated clinical scenario. Each option may be used once, more than once or not at all.

Item 1

A 20-year-old nulliparous patient at five weeks' gestation. She is on warfarin, having sustained a deep-vein thrombosis when in hospital with a fractured femur two months previously.

Item 2

A 20-year-old woman has had a normal delivery. She has been on LMWH since 30 weeks because of a deep-vein thrombosis. She wishes to breast feed and prefers not to have injections.

Item 3

A 30-year-old primigravida, BMI 21, with an uncomplicated pregnancy at 20 weeks, going on a long-haul flight from London to Auckland.

Item 4
A 25-year-old woman in her first pregnancy at 14 weeks. She is a non-smoker with a BMI of 22. She gives a history of previous deep-vein thrombosis sustained after a breast-reduction operation.

Item 5
A 38-year-old, para 4, who delivered by Caesarean section 12 hours previously.

Item 6
A 22-year-old, para 1, at eight weeks' gestation, who sustained a deep-vein thrombosis at 10 weeks in her previous pregnancy.

2   *Options*
   a   Chorionic villus sampling.
   b   A detailed fetal scan at 20 weeks.
   c   Nuchal translucency measurement and early biochemical screening.
   d   Maternal blood for chromosomes.
   e   Maternal blood for DNA testing.
   f   Paternal blood for DNA testing.

Instructions
You are required to choose the single most appropriate method of prenatal screening for each clinical scenario. Each option may be used once, more than once or not at all.

Item 1
A 28-year-old para 2 who is at eight weeks' gestation and wishes to have prenatal diagnosis to exclude cystic fibrosis. She has a child with cystic fibrosis and her husband is a carrier.

Item 2
A 40-year-old nulliparous woman who wishes to have a screening test for Down's syndrome in the first trimester.

Item 3
A 22-year-old primigravid woman at 10 weeks' gestation who has a brother with Down's syndrome and wishes to know if her pregnancy is at increased risk.

Item 4
A 32-year-old woman at eight weeks who has myotonic dystrophy and wishes to know if the pregnancy is affected.

Item 5
A 20-year-old, para 1, at eight weeks' gestation, who wishes to have prenatal testing because her child has spina bifida.

Item 6
A 32-year-old woman at seven weeks in her first pregnancy and her partner has sickle cell trait.

3 *Options*
  a Offer a membrane sweep.
  b Administer vaginal prostaglandins 3 mg.
  c Offer a Caesarean section.
  d A Caesarean section is indicated.
  e Continue conservative management.
  f Offer acupuncture or homeopathic medicine.

Instructions
You are required to choose the single most appropriate method of induction or delivery. Each option may be used once, more than once or not at all.

Item 1
Preterm prelabour rupture of membranes at 32 weeks.

Item 2
Severe intrauterine growth restriction at 35 weeks.

Item 3
Prelabour rupture of the membranes for 48 hours at 40 weeks' gestation.

Item 4
A primigravid patient at 40 weeks with an uncomplicated pregnancy.

Item 5
A parous woman who has had a previous vaginal delivery and presents with proteinuric pre-eclampsia at 38 weeks.

Item 6
An uncomplicated pregnancy at 41 weeks and five days.

4   *Options*
    a   Arrange a repeat scan at 32 weeks.
    b   Arrange a repeat scan at 36 weeks.
    c   Arrange a transvaginal scan.
    d   Arrange colour flow Doppler imaging to check for a morbidly adherent placenta.
    e   No further scans required.
    f   Arrange a repeat scan at 26 weeks.

Instructions
You are required to choose the single most appropriate option for the management of each clinical scenario relating to the management of suspected placenta praevia. Each option may be used once, more than once or not at all.

Item 1
A woman found to have a possible posterior placenta praevia at the time of her detailed scan.

Item 2
A woman who has had a previous Caesarean section and is found to have a low anterior placenta covering the internal os at 32 weeks.

Item 3
A woman found to have a low-lying placenta just reaching the internal os at the time of her detailed scan at 20 weeks and remains asymptomatic.

Item 4
A woman found to have a placenta covering the internal os at 34 weeks' gestation.

Item 5
A woman admitted with painless vaginal bleeding at 20 weeks and found to have low-lying placenta covering the internal os at the time of her detailed scan.

5   *Options*
    a   Viable intrauterine pregnancy.
    b   Missed abortion.
    c   Recurrent miscarriage.
    d   Early fetal demise.

e Pregnancy of unknown location.
f Ectopic pregnancy.
g Threatened miscarriage.
h Septic miscarriage.
i Complete miscarriage.
j Incomplete abortion.
k Blighted ovum.
l Heterotopic pregnancy.

Instructions
You are required to choose the single most appropriate clinical description of the following early-pregnancy scenarios. Each option may be used once, more than once or not at all.

Item 1
A woman presents with bleeding in early pregnancy and ultrasound scan reveals a single fetus with a crown rump length of 7 mm but no fetal heart pulsation.

Item 2
A woman presents with bleeding at five weeks and vague lower abdominal pain. The scan reveals a single fetus with a crown rump length of 2 mm and no fetal heart pulsation. A yolk sac is present.

Item 3
A woman with a history of previous ectopic pregnancy presents for scan at five weeks' gestation. The serum hCG is 1100 IU/L. The scan reveals an empty uterus with no adnexal abnormality.

Item 4
A woman presents in early pregnancy with vaginal discharge and scan reveals a single fetus with a crown rump length of 9 mm with a positive fetal heart pulsation. A vaginal swab cultures chlamydia.

Item 5
A woman presents at eight weeks' gestation with early pregnancy bleeding and a scan reveals an intrauterine sac measuring $30 \times 25 \times 28$ mm. There is no yolk sac, no fetal pole and no fetal heart pulsation.

6 *Options*
    a Perform a fetal scalp blood sample.
    b Continue to observe.
    c Perform an assisted vaginal delivery.
    d Perform an emergency Caesarean section.
    e Apply a scalp electrode.

Instructions
You are required to choose the single most appropriate option for the management of each fetal heart rate pattern. The woman has had an uncomplicated pregnancy and is in spontaneous labour with a vertex presentation in her second pregnancy. She had a previous normal delivery. Each option may be used once, more than once or not at all.

Item 1
A fetal heart rate baseline of 170 beats per minute with normal variability for the past 30 minutes. There are no decelerations, and accelerations are present. The cervix is 5 cm dilated.

Item 2
A fetal heart rate baseline of 140 beats with reduced variability for 100 minutes. There are occasional late decelerations. The cervix is 3 cm dilated and there is meconium-stained amniotic fluid.

Item 3
A fetal heart rate baseline of 165 beats per minute with normal variability. Over the past 30 minutes variable decelerations have appeared. The cervix is 8 cm dilated.

Item 4
A fetal heart rate baseline which has dropped from 140 beats per minute to 70 beats per minute for the last 10 minutes. The patient has been fully dilated for 120 minutes and the vertex is in the occipito-posterior position, stationed 1 cm above the spines.

Item 5
A fetal heart rate baseline of 115 beats per minute with normal variability. There have been atypical variable decelerations for 60 minutes and the cervix is 7 cm dilated.

7 *Options*

   a No risk.
   b 1 in 2.
   c 1 in 3.
   d 1 in 4.
   e 1 in 20.
   f 1 in 50.
   g 1 in 500.
   h 1 in 1000.
   i 1 in 2000.
   j 1 in 5000.

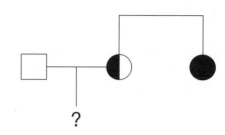

Instructions

You are seeing a Caucasian couple from Edinburgh for pre-pregnancy counselling. The wife, whose sister has cystic fibrosis, is known to be a carrier for the cystic fibrosis gene. The husband has not been tested. They wish to know some facts about their risks of having an affected child. Each option may be used once, more than once or not at all.

Item 1

They wish to know the incidence of cystic fibrosis in their population.

Item 2

The husband wishes to know his risk of being a carrier.

Item 3

If he does not carry an identifiable mutation, what is the risk of the child being affected?

Item 4

If he was found to be a carrier for cystic fibrosis, what is the risk of the offspring being affected?

Item 5

If they have an affected child, what will be the risk of having a second affected child?

8 *Options*

a No risk.

b 1 in 1.

c 1 in 2.

d 1 in 3.

e 1 in 4.

f 1 in 20.

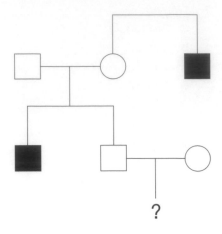

Instructions

You are seeing a healthy couple at the antenatal clinic at 10 weeks' gestation. When enquiring about any family history the husband mentions that he has a brother and an uncle on his mother's side with mental retardation due to fragile X. He has been told that it is a genetic disorder. He works as a school teacher. They wish to know some facts about their risks of having an affected child. Each option may be used once, more than once or not at all.

Item 1

What is the husband's risk of being a carrier for mental retardation?

Item 2

If he was a carrier for the most common single gene disorder for mental retardation, what would be the risk of a male child carrying the gene?

Item 3

If he was a carrier for the most common single gene disorder for mental retardation, what would be the risk of a female child carrying the gene?

Item 4

What are the chances that his mother is a carrier of the gene?

Item 5

What are the chances that his father is a carrier of the affected gene?

9 *Options*

   a No risk.

   b 1 in 2.

   c 1 in 3.

   d 1 in 4.

   e 1 in 8.

   f 1 in 10.

   g 1 in 100.

   h 1 in 200.

   i 1 in 500.

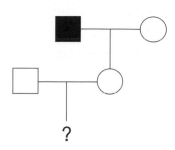

Instructions

You are asked to see a pregnant woman at eight weeks' gestation. Her father has Huntington's disease. You are required to give the risk estimates for each of the following questions asked by the patient. Each option may be used once, more than once or not at all.

Item 1

What is the risk of her developing Huntington's disease?

Item 2

What is the risk of her unborn child developing the disease if he was male?

Item 3

She wishes to have testing by chorionic villus sampling at 11 weeks. What is the risk of miscarriage from the procedure?

Item 4

She enquires about fetal exclusion testing that will give the risk to the fetus without predicting her genetic status. What will be the risk to the fetus of inheriting a chromosome from her father?

Item 5

If both she and her husband were carriers for Huntington's disease, what would be the chance of having an unaffected child?

10 *Options*

    a Offer chorionic villus sampling.

    b Neonatal follow-up scans.

    c Offer termination of pregnancy.

    d Repeat the scan in three weeks' time.

    e Ask paediatric surgical consultant to counsel.

    f Offer fetal blood sampling.

    g Offer amniocentesis.

    h Insert a shunt.

Instructions

Each of the following clinical scenarios relates to management of a fetal abnormality. Choose the single most appropriate option. Each option may be used once, more than once or not at all.

Item 1

Bilateral renal pelvic dilatation seen at a detailed scan at 20 weeks. There is no other detected abnormality.

Item 2

Anencephaly at 12 weeks.

Item 3

Spina bifida with hydrocephaly.

Item 4

Midgut herniation at 11 weeks.

Item 5

Exomphalos at 20 weeks.

Item 6

Gastroschisis at 20 weeks.

11 *Options*
  a Advise against air travel.
  b Advise to wear graduated elastic compression stockings.
  c Advise to wear graduated elastic compression stockings and to take low-dose aspirin.
  d Advise to wear graduated elastic compression stockings and to have thromboprophylaxis with low molecular weight heparin.
  e Advise that no specific measures required.

Instructions
Each of the following clinical scenarios relates to advice on air travel and pregnancy. Choose the single most appropriate option. Each option may be used once, more than once or not at all.

Item 1
A 35-year-old woman in her first pregnancy with an uncomplicated singleton pregnancy at 20 weeks' gestation going on a two-hour flight.

Item 2
A 25-year-old para 1 having had a previous uncomplicated pregnancy going on a four-hour flight at 38 weeks. This pregnancy has been uncomplicated.

Item 3
A 20-year-old primigravida with a body mass index of 36 with an uncomplicated pregnancy at 26 weeks' gestation going on a three-hour flight.

Item 4
An 18-year-old primigravida with an uncomplicated pregnancy at 26 weeks' pregnancy going on an eight-hour flight.

Item 5
A 32-year-old primigravida with an uncomplicated twin pregnancy at 36 weeks' gestation going on a three-hour flight.

12 *Options*

    a Anticipate spontaneous vaginal delivery.

    b Perform mid-cavity forceps delivery.

    c Perform vacuum or mid-cavity forceps delivery.

    d Perform lower-segment Caesarean section.

    e Perform classical Caesarean section.

    f Perform episiotomy.

    g Perform rotational forceps or vacuum delivery.

    h Give syntocinon.

Instructions

Each of the following clinical scenarios relates to the management of the second stage of labour. Choose the single most appropriate option. Each option may be used once, more than once or not at all.

Item 1

A para 4 at term with a mento-posterior face presentation at 0 + 1 station who has been fully dilated for two hours.

Item 2

A primiparous woman at term who is hepatitis C positive and has been fully dilated for one hour.

Item 3

A primiparous woman at 33 weeks who has been fully dilated for two hours and has been pushing for the previous one hour with a vertex presentation, occipito-posterior position, stationed 2 cm below the ischial spines.

Item 4

A primiparous patient at term with a vertex presentation in the occipito position, stationed 1 cm below the ischial spines. She has been fully dilated for one hour and has an epidural. The contractions have reduced to one in five minutes.

Item 5

A parous woman at term who has had two previous normal deliveries and has been fully dilated for one hour. The vertex is in the occipito-anterior position, stationed 1 cm below the spines, and there have been atypical variable decelerations for 30 minutes.

13 *Options*
- a Dichorionic diamniotic.
- b Monochorionic diamniotic.
- c Monochorionic monoamniotic.
- d Subchorionic haematoma in a dichorionic twin pregnancy.
- e Twin-to-twin transfusion.
- f Growth discordancy.

Instructions
Each of the following ultrasound reports relate to chorionicity and twin pregnancy. Choose the single most appropriate option. Each option may be used once, more than once or not at all.

Item 1
An ultrasound scan at 12 weeks shows a twin pregnancy with the presence of a lambda sign.

Item 2
An ultrasound scan at 32 weeks in a dichorionic twin pregnancy shows a 30 mm difference in the abdominal circumference of each twin.

Item 3
An ultrasound scan at 12 weeks shows a twin pregnancy with the presence of a T sign.

Item 4
An ultrasound scan in a monochorionic twin pregnancy shows a 30 mm difference in the abdominal circumference of each twin.

Item 5
An ultrasound scan at 15 weeks shows a twin pregnancy with no dividing membrane between each sac.

Item 6
An ultrasound scan at 12 weeks shows a twin pregnancy with one chorion and a single yolk sac.

14 *Options*

    a Admit to hospital for further assessment.

    b Manage in community and perform full blood count and liver function tests.

    c Manage in community without any blood tests.

    d Admit to hospital for immediate induction.

    e Commence antihypertensive treatment.

Instructions

Each of the following relates to the management of pregnancy-associated hypertension. You are assessing each patient in the antenatal clinic. Choose the single most appropriate option. Each option may be used once, more than once or not at all.

Item 1

A 32-year-old primigravida with a booking blood pressure of 150/100 at 12 weeks and no proteinuria.

Item 2

A 32-year-old para 1 with a previous uncomplicated pregnancy at 37 weeks' gestation with a blood pressure of 130/90 and proteinuria ++++.

Item 3

A 24-year-old primigravida at 32 weeks with a blood pressure of 140/85 and no proteinuria.

Item 4

A 22-year-old primigravida at 28 weeks' gestation with a blood pressure of 140/90 and proteinuria +.

Item 5

An 18-year-old primigravida at 26 weeks with a blood pressure of 160/100 and no proteinuria.

15 *Options*
   a Give anti-D 250 IU minimum.
   b Give anti-D 500 IU minimum.
   c Do not give anti-D.
   d Give anti-D 500 IU and check for fetal maternal haemorrhage.
   e Check Rhesus blood group of father.

Instructions
Each of the following relates to the need for administration of anti-D immunoglobulin. Choose the single most appropriate option. Each option may be used once, more than once or not at all.

Item 1
A non-sensitised Rhesus-negative woman who has had a salpingectomy for an ectopic pregnancy.

Item 2
A non-sensitised Rhesus-negative woman who has had a medical termination of pregnancy at eight weeks' gestation.

Item 3
A non-sensitised Rhesus-negative woman who has had a spontaneous miscarriage at eight weeks' gestation.

Item 4
A non-sensitised Rhesus-negative woman who has a threatened miscarriage at 22 weeks' gestation.

Item 5
A non-sensitised Rhesus-negative woman who has delivered a Rhesus-positive baby.

Item 6
A non-sensitised Rhesus-negative woman who has a Rhesus-positive husband and has delivered a Rhesus-negative baby.

Answers: EMQs: obstetrics

1   1d, 2h, 3f, 4e, 5a, 6a.

2   1a, 2c, 3d, 4a, 5b, 6e.

3   1e, 2d, 3b, 4a, 5b, 6b.
    (Reference: NICE guideline 70. Induction of labour, 2008.)

4   1c, 2d, 3b, 4b, 5f.
    (Reference: RCOG guideline 27. Placenta praevia and placenta praevia accreta: diagnosis and management.)

5   1d, 2g, 3e, 4a, 5d.
    (Reference: RCOG greentop guideline 25. Management of early pregnancy loss.)

6   1b, 2d, 3a, 4d, 5a.
    (Reference: NICE guideline on use and interpretation of cardiotocography, 2001.)

7   1i, 2e, 3g, 4d, 5d.
    Cystic fibrosis is an autosomal-recessive condition with a 1 in 4 risk to the offspring if each parent is a carrier. It is the most common autosomal-recessive disorder in northern Europeans, with 1 in 20 of the population being carriers, resulting in 1 in 2000 live births being affected. Screening for the four most common cystic fibrosis mutations in northern Europeans identifies 85% of carriers.

8   1c, 2a, 3b, 4b, 5a.
    This question relates to fragile X syndrome, which is the commonest cause of severe mental retardation after Down's syndrome, affecting around 1 in 2000 individuals. It is inherited as an X-linked trait and so males in the family will be affected. Half the sons of a carrier female will be affected and all the daughters of a male will be carriers. However, it is more complicated. Due to the nature of the fragile X mutation, female carriers may be affected and apparently unaffected males (normal transmitting males) may have the gene. The husband in this scenario could be a normal transmitting male.

9 1b, 2d, 3g, 4b, 5d.

Huntington's disease is an autosomal-dominant condition, meaning that there is a 1 in 2 risk of inheritance. The patient does not know if she is a carrier and so the risk to the fetus is 1 in 4. Chorion biopsy has a procedure-related loss rate of 1 in 50 to 1 in 100. The defective gene is on chromosome 4. The fetus has a 1 in 2 risk of inheriting chromosome 4 from her father. The information on whether it is the affected or unaffected chromosome is not tested for, because the pregnant woman does not wish to know that fact. If she and her husband carried the gene, the risks are that one child would have both genes, two would have one gene and one would be lucky.

10 1b, 2c, 3c, 4d, 5g, 6e.

11 1e, 2a, 3d, 4b, 5a.

(Reference: RCOG Scientific Advisory Committee Opinion paper on Air Travel in Pregnancy.)

12 1d, 2a, 3b, 4h, 5c.

13 1a, 2f, 3b, 4e, 5c, 6c.

14 1e, 2d, 3c, 4b, 5a.

(Reference: RCOG guideline 10. The management of severe pre-eclampsia/eclampsia.)

15 1a, 2a, 3c, 4b, 5d, 6c.

(Reference: RCOG guideline 22. Use of anti-D immunoglobulin for Rh prophylaxis.)

Extended matching questions: gynaecology

1 a renal colic
  b threatened miscarriage
  c acute appendicitis
  d hepatitis
  e ulcerative colitis
  f ectopic pregnancy
  g Meckel's diverticulum
  h diverticulosis
  i pelvic inflammatory disease
  j Crohn's disease
  k torted ovarian cyst
  l hydrosalpinges
  m haematometra
  n cholecystitis
  o irritable bowel syndrome

For each clinical scenario below give the most likely diagnosis from the list above. Each diagnosis may be used only once.

1 A 29-year-old woman presents with six weeks' amenorrhoea, some vaginal bleeding and pain in the right iliac fossa.

2 A 19-year-old woman presents with right iliac fossa pain, irregular periods on the mini pill, fever and anorexia.

3 A 42-year-old woman presents with bilateral lower abdominal pain, fever and a vaginal discharge.

4 A 24-year-old woman presents with regular periods, cramping, diffuse abdominal pain associated with constipation and diarrhoea.

5 A 40-year-old woman with regular periods presents with continuous right upper quadrant pain, vomiting and fever. She is tender in the right upper quadrant.

6 A 36-year-old woman presents with three months' amenorrhoea, weight loss, diarrhoea and abdominal pain and iron deficiency. Pregnancy test is negative.

7 A 30-year-old woman presents with regular periods and sudden onset of colicky left iliac fossa pain. She is very tender on the left with rebound and has cervical excitation.

8 A 35-year-old woman presents with six months' amenorrhoea, cyclical pelvic pain and a history of a cervical cone biopsy seven months ago.

2 a oestrogen
 b progesterone
 c testosterone
 d inhibin
 e FSH
 f LH
 g oestrogen and progesterone

Name the hormone or hormone combination (as in g) that causes the effects described below (each answer can be used more than once).

1 This hormone rises if oestrogen levels fall.

2 proliferation of breast tissue at puberty

3 endometrial proliferation

4 at puberty causes closure of the long bone ephiphyses

5 limits pre-partum lactation

6 pubic and axillary hair growth

7 thick cervical mucous production

8 maturation of vaginal epithelium

9 sexual differentiation in the fetus

10 inhibits FSH secretion

3 a atrophic endometrium
   b secretory endometrium
   c proliferative endometrium
   d adenocarcinoma
   e cystic hyperplasia
   f decidual reaction
   g hydropic vesicles
   h simple hyperplasia
   i transitional cell carcinoma

The following women have had endometrial biopsies taken. Please match the most likely histology of the endometrium from the list above to the clinical scenario described below. Each histological diagnosis can be used only once.

1 A 58-year-old obese diabetic woman presents with postmenopausal bleeding over the past six months. LMP – 12 years ago. The transvaginal scan (TVS) shows an endometrial thickness of 15 mm.

2 A 58-year-old woman has just commenced continuous combined HRT three months ago and has had some vaginal bleeding. LMP – two years ago. The TVS shows an endometrial thickness of 2 mm.

3 A 32-year-old woman has four years of infertility with regular 32-day cycles. An endometrial biopsy is taken on day 26.

4 A 24-year-old woman presents with a ruptured ectopic pregnancy of six weeks' gestation. During the laparoscopy curettage is performed.

5 A 26-year-old woman presents with eight weeks' amenorrhoea, a positive pregnancy test and vaginal bleeding. The TVS shows a 'snowstorm' appearance. She goes to the operating theatre for an evacuation.

6 A 54-year-old woman has been on unopposed oestrogen therapy for 18 months and had one episode of vaginal bleeding. The TVS showed endometrial thickness of 8 mm.

7 A 54-year-old woman is taking cyclical transdermal HRT. She is having regular withdrawal bleeds but is concerned

regarding family history of endometrial cancer. She had an endometrial biopsy taken on day eight of the cycle.

4 a stress incontinence
  b urinary tract infection
  c urge incontinence
  d neuropathic bladder
  e carcinoma of the bladder
  f urethral diverticulum
  g rectocele
  h cystocele
  i procidentia
  j vesicovaginal fistula

Match the most likely diagnosis from the list above with the clinical scenarios described below. Each diagnosis can be used only once.

1 A 46-year-old woman had a vaginal hysterectomy, anterior and posterior repair performed six weeks ago and has been complaining of a persistent watery discharge that has the characteristics of urine.

2 A 40-year-old woman complains of a one-week history of dysuria, frequency and nocturia.

3 A 38-year-old woman complains of a 'lump' in the anterior vagina and sometimes has a urethral discharge.

4 A 40-year-old woman complains of a 12-month history of urinary urgency, dysuria, frequency and nocturia.

5 A 60-year-old woman complains of a 'bulge' down below and has to put a finger into the vagina to be able to evacuate her bowel.

6 A 45-year-old woman presents with a three-month history of haematuria.

7 A 40-year-old woman complains of a 12-month history of urinary incontinence when she laughs or coughs.

5   Theme: diagnostic and screening tests
    a   accuracy
    b   disease negative
    c   false positive
    d   likelihood ratio of positive test
    e   negative predictive value
    f   numbers needed to treat
    g   odds ratio
    h   *p* value
    i   positive predictive value
    j   sensitivity
    k   specificity
    l   true negative

For each of the questions below, choose the item that provides the answer from the above list of options. Each option may be used once, more than once or not at all.

    1   How good is this test at correctly excluding people without the condition?
    2   What is the term for individuals who do not have the condition yet have a positive test result?
    3   What proportion of individuals with the condition are detected by the test?
    4   If a person has a negative test, what is the probability that he/she does not have the condition?
    5   Who has a negative test result and does not have the condition?

6   a   androgen-binding protein (ABP)
    b   dihydrate testosterone (DHT)
    c   oestradiol 17β
    d   follicle-stimulating hormone (FSH)
    e   gonadotrophin-releasing hormone (GnRH)
    f   growth hormone (GH)
    g   inhibin
    h   luteinising hormone (LH)
    i   melatonin
    j   testosterone

Regarding testosterone function, match the description below with one of the hormones above. The hormones above can be used only once.

1 The hormone produced by the anterior pituitary that acts on Sertoli cells.

2 The hormone produced by the anterior pituitary that acts on Leydig cells.

3 The hormone produced by the Leydig cells.

4 A hormone produced by Sertoli cells that can potentiate Leydig cell function.

5 The hormone released by the hypothalamus that acts on the anterior pituitary.

7 a gonadotrophin-releasing hormone
b luteinising hormone
c follicle-stimulating hormone
d oestradiol
e progesterone
f androstenedione
g inhibin
h prolactin
i growth hormone
j cholesterol

Regarding female reproductive endocrinology, please match the description below with a hormone above. Each hormone can be used only once.

1 Is produced by the thecal cells of the Graafian follicle and is used as a precursor for follicular oestradiol synthesis.

2 Stimulates oestradiol secretion from the corpus luteum.

3 Is responsible for feedback onto the hypothalamic pituitary axis to initiate the pre-ovulatary LH surge.

4 Is secreted by hypothalamic neurons.

5 Selectively suppresses FSH production.

6 Is raised in women who have galactorrhoea.

7 Peaks in the middle of the secretory phase of the menstrual cycle.

8   a ectopic pregnancy
    b cystic hyperplasia
    c haematometra
    d molar pregnancy
    e calcified serosal fibroid
    f calcified intramural fibroid
    g pseudosac
    h intrauterine sac
    i displaced IUCD

You are required to match the following pictures with the most appropriate scan findings as above.

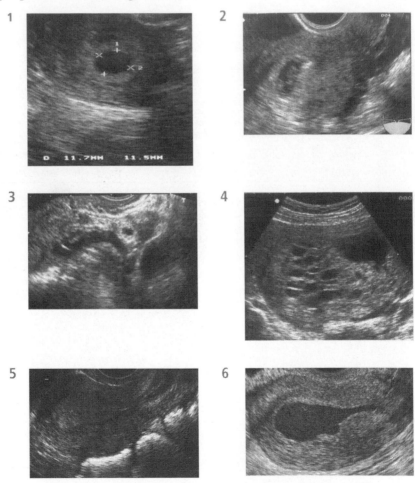

7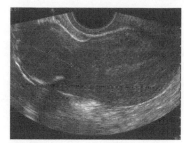

8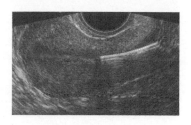

9 a 1.0–1.5
  b 4.0–5.5
  c 0.1–1.0
  d 0.3–3.0
  e 0.1–1.2
  f 0.5–2.0
  g 0.13
  h 0.02
  i 4–25
  j 0.1

Match the contraceptive method with the most accurate failure rate per 100 women years. Each failure rate may be used only once.

	failure rate per 100 women years
1 injectables	
2 female sterilisation	
3 progestogen-only oral contraceptives	
4 copper IUDs	
5 progestogen IUS	
6 diaphragm	
7 male sterilisation	
8 implants	
9 withdrawal	

10 a infertility
  b vaginal cancer
  c cervical cancer
  d endometrial cancer
  e ovarian cancer
  f vulval cancer
  g fallopian tube cancer

Match the following risk factors with the above conditions. Each condition may be used once, more than once or not at all.

  1 nulliparity and obesity

  2 smoking and low socioeconomic status

  3 talcum powder

  4 chlamydial infection

  5 ruptured appendix

  6 BRCAI gene

11 a hysteroscopy
  b colposcopy
  c TAH and BSO
  d operative hysteroscopy
  e oral contraceptive pill
  f tranexamic acid
  g operative laparoscopy
  h endocervical swabs
  i cryotherapy
  j hysterectomy
  k myomectomy

With the following scenarios choose the most appropriate management from the list above. Each option may be used once only.

  1 A 16-year-old girl with heavy painful periods.

  2 A 40-year-old woman with heavy periods and a submucosal fibroid.

  3 A 40-year-old woman with painful periods, a right-sided 4 cm ovarian cyst and a CA125 of 65.

4   An inflammatory smear in a 24-year-old.

5   A woman with post-coital bleeding who has had two normal smears but has an ectropion.

6   A 30-year-old woman who has a smear showing moderate dyskaryosis.

12 a   risidronate

   b   oestradiol

   c   progestogens

   d   venlafaxine

   e   dalacin cream

   f   premarin cream

   g   microgynon

   h   tranexamic acid

   i   mefenamic acid

   j   carbergoline

   k   tolteridine

   l   tibolone

   m   tamoxifen

   n   metformin

   o   dianette

For each of the following conditions select the most appropriate drug treatment from the list above. Each drug cannot be used more than once.

1   A 30-year-old woman is prescribed Zoladex for 12 months to suppress her endometriosis. She needs an agent to protect against bone loss and relieve her hypo-oestrogenic symptoms.

2   A 55-year-old woman is having dreadful hot flushes but will not take HRT.

3   A 26-year-old woman has galactorrhoea, a raised serum prolactin and amenorrhoea.

4   A 35-year-old woman has heavy regular periods.

5   A 40-year-old woman has tried metronidozole for her bacterial vaginosis but it has not worked.

6   A 30-year-old woman has hirsuitism and oligoamenorrhoea and is known to have PCOS.

13 a PMT symptoms
b dry mouth
c nausea and abdominal discomfort
d rise in liver enzymes
e breast discomfort
f hot flushes
g breakthrough bleeding
h urticaria
i oily skin

Match the side effects from the list above that occur with the following medications. The side effects can be used once, more than once or not at all.

1 fluconazole

2 HRT

3 progestogen-only pill

4 metformin

5 oxybutynin

6 danazol

7 progestogens

8 GnRH analogues

9 cyproterone acetate

10 tamoxifen

11 Mirena

14 a increased LH, normal FSH, normal oestradiol
b increased LH, increased FSH, low oestradiol
c decreased LH, decreased FSH, low oestradiol
d increased LH, increased FSH, normal oestradiol
e normal LH, normal FSH, normal oestradiol

Match the most appropriate hormone profile from the list above with each condition below. Each profile can be used once, more than once or not at all.

1 anorexia nervosa

2 postmenopausal not on HRT

3 postmenopausal on HRT

4 PCOS

5 excessive exercise and amenorrhoea

6 25-year-old with premature ovarian failure

15 a intracytoplasmic sperm injection
   b *in vitro* fertilisation
   c gamete intrafallopian transfer
   d intrauterine insemination
   e artificial insemination by donor
   f clomiphene
   g ovum donation
   h artificial insemination from husband

From the list above choose the most appropriate management for the conditions below. Each management can be used only once.

1 bilateral tubal blockage

2 premature ovarian failure

3 azoospermia

4 PCOS

5 partner with paraplegia

6 unexplained infertility for five years

Answers: EMQs: gynaecology

1
1	f	2	c	3	i	4	o
5	n	6	j	7	k	8	m

2
1	e	2	g	3	a	4	c
5	b	6	c	7	b	8	a
9	c	10	d				

3
1	d	2	a	3	b	4	f
5	g	6	h	7	c		

4
1	j	2	b	3	f	4	c
5	h	6	e	7	a		

5
1	k	2	c	3	j	4	e
5	l						

6
1	d	2	h	3	j	4	g
5	e						

7
1	f	2	c	3	d	4	a
5	g	6	h	7	e		

8
1	h	2	g	3	a	4	d
5	b	6	c	7	e	8	i

9
1	e	2	g	3	d	4	f
5	j	6	a	7	h	8	o
9	i						

10
1	d	2	c	3	e	4	a
5	a	6	e				

11
1	e	2	d	3	g	4	h
5	i	6	b				

12
1	l	2	d	3	j	4	h
5	e	6	o				

13
1	c	2	e	3	g	4	c
5	b	6	i	7	a	8	f
9	d	10	f	11	g		

14 1 c   2 b   3 d   4 a
     5 c   6 b

15 1 b   2 g   3 e   4 f
     5 a   6 b

Index